THE SCIENCE OF MEDICAL ASTROLOGY

THE EXPERIMENTAL PROOF OF JYOTISHA

I0396770

RAMESHRAO N.
ALEX HANKEY

INDICACADEMY

notionpress.com

INDIA • SINGAPORE • MALAYSIA

Notion Press

Old No. 38, New No. 6
McNichols Road, Chetpet
Chennai - 600 031

First Published by Notion Press 2019

ISBN 978-1-64783-643-6

CONTENTS

Preface 5

1. Introduction 7

2. Overview of the Experiments
   Strengths and Weaknesses 17

3. Vaccination Experiments 23

4. Bacterial Vaccine Production 37

5. Viral Vaccine Production Experiments 45

6. Solar Eclipse Experiments 53

7. A Physical Theory of Astrology 59

8. Discussion and Conclusions 73

Epilogue

The Nature of Time 89

Appendix

Concept of Environment according to Vedas: Vāstu 93

PREFACE

In 2013, my unique PhD student, Dr Rameshrao, graduated after conducting revolutionary research on *Jyotisha* astrology. Confounding scientific prejudice, his experiments met with success. Their extraordinary results converted many from disbelief into acceptance.

I met Rameshrao on my first day at S-VYASA in September 2007, after being taken by Vice-Chancellor Nagendra to meet prospective research students. Research proposals were considered and accepted. Only Rameshrao's met disapproval. The reason, "No one on faculty understands *Jyotisha,* so we cannot supervise your proposal." Immediately I said, "I know *Jyotisha* well. I have studied it for 20 years and would be happy to advise him."

Everyone looked at me suspiciously. How could a physicist trained at Cambridge and M.I.T. know Indian, *Jyotisha* astrology? But it was true. I had worked for Maharishi Mahesh Yogi for 30 years and learned much about *Jyotisha* astrology. In 1988, I attended a course in New Delhi, which introduced us to *Jyotisha* as a tool to diagnose health weaknesses. At that time, I drew up my *Kundali* birth-chart.

My birth certificate told the address, *Dharma Court* in Oxted, England, but not my birth time. My widowed father told me that I had been born while he was at work, limiting me to five possible rising signs. Despite my lack of experience, the clue enabled me to select *Thula,* Libra in *Jyotisha.* Later, when professionals 'rectified' my chart, that turned out to be correct. Duly impressed, I had read several books, gaining familiarity and trust in the system, but not real expertise in its practice. In 2004, I expressed serious interest in conducting research on it to a close academic friend who encouraged me.

Meeting Ramesh fulfilled this desire. His 3-month experiment on vaccination of sheep and goats was planned to start in December 2007. It would assess vaccinated animals after three and thirteen weeks. Unfortunately, the experiment was ruined by a storm later that winter, when many sheep died. The final data was deficient. Initial analysis suggested some good effects, but not the kind of power expected for a PhD. A further experiment on a different breed of sheep at another farm was undertaken in August, 2008, but problems of publishing results in a scientific journal were too challenging. Only later did we find a means of data analysis that yielded good results (see Chapter 3).

In 2011, Ramesh persuaded senior colleagues at the Institute for Animal Health and Veterinary Biology producing Karnataka's veterinary vaccines to conduct experiments on vaccine production. The vaccine against Blue Tongue disease that decimates flocks of sheep and goats was selected. Vaccine production runs starting at times considered 'auspicious' and 'inauspicious' were assessed.

The experiment's success led to many more. All produced highly significant results. Many were published. Rameshrao's discoveries are revolutionary for biology, medical science, and *Jyotisha* astrology itself. They are the most significant that I have witnessed first-hand. I have even developed a new theory of the physics involved, related in the book. I wish readers an enthralling read.

Chapter 1

INTRODUCTION

Are you fascinated by the idea of astrology? That the positions of the planets might somehow correlate with events in our lives? If they influence human life, do you suppose that they might affect other living things? This little book gives a short account of a series of experiments conclusively demonstrating that planets are affecting life everywhere. Every cell in every living organism on Planet Earth is continuously being guided by influences correlated with the positions of the sun and moon, the planets, and other aspects of the sky around us.

How could this be, you may ask? If you are a scientist, the idea may seem outrageous, too shocking to consider. That the authors are scientists with over 70 years' experience of teaching and research between them, and both convinced of the value and validity of science and scientific methods, might also seem confusing. Yet it is true. Turn the pages of this book to find out why, and how the experiments were performed. See if you too are not convinced.

The aim of the book is to give some grounding in India's system of *Jyotisha* astrology, the first author's personal perspective on it, and the experiments that he designed. *Jyotisha* is a sidereal system of astrology, meaning that the astrological signs are fixed to the positions of the stars in the sky, and do not rotate with the precession of the equinoxes. Its roots can be traced to the beginning of the Vedic system of knowledge, over 8,000 years ago. It is an integral aspect of the Vedic sciences, being the last of the six *Vedangas*, the 'limbs of the Vedas'.

The first author has spent a quarter-century assessing *Jyotisha* questions after work on weekday evenings. That, combined with his profession as a veterinary scientist working for India's state of Karnataka, has given him a unique understanding of the whole field. He likes to present a scientific perspective on *Jyotisha* as a manifestation of the inner force of nature, similar to light, which gives all nature manifestation. This chapter introduces his perspective on *Jyotisha*; Chapters 2 to 6 tell the story of the experiments. Chapter 7 outlines a vision of the second author's physical theory of what makes *Jyotisha* possible; Chapter 8 presents conclusions.

Central to astrology is the idea that the sun, moon and planets can influence peoples' minds and other tendencies that make events happen in biological and physical worlds here on earth. *Jyotisha* includes two other non-luminous bodies as well, the nodes of the moon, called *Rahu* and *Ketu*, explained in more detail below. Equally important are the ideas that some of these *grahas*, as *Jyotisha* calls them, have intrinsically benefic properties, and that times when their influence is strong are 'auspicious'. Other *grahas* have intrinsically malefic properties, and times when their influence is strong are 'inauspicious'. For example, if someone wins a lottery, or receives recognition for their hard work and achievements, that will come from the influence of a benefic planet. On the other hand, if they have an accident and end up in hospital, that will be associated with the malign influence of a malefic planet. Such events would obviously be regarded as 'auspicious' and 'inauspicious' respectively.

The most important point about the experiments is that the results were self-consistent and mutually supportive. Self-consistency is important; it provides a further level of validation of *Jyotisha* concepts, beyond that of each experiment by itself; further reason to think that the results were not obtained by chance, and that more research is merited. Chapter 8 summarizes the many discoveries made by the research, showing particularly how the concepts of benefic and malefic, and auspicious and inauspicious, were given precise meaning in terms of influence on immune response, bacterial growth (the two most elaborate experiments), and viral propagation, another six experiments. The theoretical physics used in the theory described in layman's terms in chapter 7 is significant. It does not just describe influences of planets on cells on earth. Its principles show how astrology may apply on the sun and other planets in the solar system, indeed, in all planetary systems.

Finally, a word about the methods used to analyse the experiments: all scientific experiments must be repeatable, but no two experiments can be expected to give identical results. Statistics are therefore required to analyse each experiment, or series of experiments. Each experiment is designed to test one or more 'experimental hypotheses'. Philosophy of science calls them 'conjectures'. Hopefully, statistical analyses of data support conjectures that an experiment was designed to test. Here, each experiment validated its experimental hypothesis with excellent statistical significance. Each stands firm in its own ground. Taken all together, results are impressive. Seldom, has a PhD yielded such a wealth of discoveries and scientific advances.

1.1 Some Background

The first author, who instigated the research, learned *Jyotisha* astrology in hospital, while he was recovering from a near-fatal accident that occurred on the very day predicted by *Jyotisha*. Not having believed a word of the prediction, he became a sincere student of the ancient science, and studied the field thoroughly during the three years that it took him to recover. He now offers his understanding to all who come to him. Thousands call every year seeking means to overcome problems they face. Many profound stories can be told. But turning the pages of this book tells an even more remarkable story than anecdotes, charming as such tales may be.

Here, for the first time, predictions of *Jyotisha* astrology are shown to be scientifically testable; and in experiments not involving people, but cells. The experiments reflect the inner nature of astrology as a discipline that can be adapted to requirements of experiment. Veterinary microbiologists from top scientific institutions demonstrated this, as we relate.

More important is the metaphysical background of *Jyotisha*. Trained scientists see the world as manifesting orderly functioning originating in deep underlying principles. Such principles lie behind the obvious Laws of Nature observed in the world around us. The Vedic *Rishis*, leaders of India's ancient Vedic civilisation, called them '*Devata*', impulses of divine intelligence that give structure, guidance and meaning to all life's experiences. Their organising power is responsible for the orderliness observed in Nature, and our power to perceive and interpret it.

The *Rishis* saw the full range of cosmic creative intelligence as '*Anoraniyan Mahatomahiyan*', from 'The Smaller than the Smallest to the Larger than the Largest'. The same is true of those at the forefront of modern mathematical physics, who hold to Einstein's vision, that all phenomena in the universe are describable by a perfectly integrated structure of Natural Law. That integrated structure can command and regulate all activities on all scales of existence, especially all levels of biological regulation. From the perspective of *Jyotisha,* astrological mediation of the planets is the means by which this integrated structure is achieved. They reach into the biochemical and biophysical regulation of man's body, mind and soul. By biophysical planetary influences outlined in Chapter 7, Cosmic Creative Intelligence can bridge all levels of gross manifestation. From its high plane of cognition of the total structure of creation, it transmits its influence into single cells, be they microbes living in apparent separation and isolation from each other, or cells in the tissues of some higher, multicellular organism.

Each of us can experience such influences as vibratory qualities influencing tendencies of mind at each point in time; qualities that act like coloured spectacles, influencing the way we experience and evaluate the world around us. The Vedic *Rishis* trained people in means to become more sensitive to subtle levels of mind where such colours can be clearly experienced.

In the second author's case, regular practice of deep meditation made him sensitive to those subtle qualities of experience; vibratory qualities that underlie all other experiences in life, both mental and sensory. Those vibratory qualities, rather like those in the rainbow, can colour our lives in personal ways, characterizing different time-periods of our lives. In that sense, they appear subjective. When associated with the physical location of a planet, they are objective.

At any given time, a person is under the guiding influence of many planets, or *grahas* in the words of *Jyotisha.* Each *graha* influences a person's life for a specific period of time, called its *Dasha* period. The sequence of nine *Dasha* periods totals 120 years, held by *Jyotisha* to be the natural length of a healthy life.

Each *Dasha* period is divided into nine subperiods of the same proportions, starting with the same *graha.* This sequence applies to further subdivisions. The *Dasha* periods endow *Jyotisha* with power to make accurate, time specific, predictions. One sequence of *Dasha* periods depending on the moon's natal position influences the mind. Another sequence, depending on the natal *Lagna* position, influences the body. *Jyotisha* cycles are structured internally; they complement circadian rhythms caused by external influences.

Increased personal sensitivity makes one aware of such influences on feelings and thoughts. *Jyotisha* influences resulting in obvious physiological changes include: (1) Entry into a new *Dasha* period; (2) Qualities of different *pakshas,* lunar fortnights, the *Shukla Paksha,* when the moon is waxing, and the *Krishna Paksha* when it is waning; the transition from one to the other is felt almost immediately after *Chandra* crosses the point of Full Moon. (3) Changes of state of the most powerful *grahas, Surya,* the Sun, *Chandra,* the moon, and the two *grahas,* Jupiter, *Guru,* and Saturn, *Shani. Jyotisha* texts use the word '*Grahasputa*' to describe subtle feelings connected to *Grahas.* The *Rishis* of *Jyotisha,* describe them in terms that we too recognise.

Our sensitivity to these subtle influences, whether consciously recognised or unrecognised, is universal – it is a Law of Nature emerging from *Jyotisha.* The influences lead us to conclude that we should adopt correct values towards the Supreme Ruler of the universe, the 'Light'. We live in the Shelter of that Light. The Womb of the Light, the manifesting power of the universe, contains seven colours. Each is like a Language of Nature expressing itself like a Thread of Music, with power to transform feelings and emotions by its influence; a stimulating force that guides manufacture of biomolecules such as chains of amino acid polypeptides bound into protein enzymes, for the manufacture of hormones, carbohydrates and lipids, and the all-important nucleic acids. All depend on regulation processes in modern complexity biology, which, as we later suggest, are guided by *Jyotisha.*

From such a perspective, the Cosmos seems highly intelligent, reaching down into the hearts of its creatures to guide them all. Based on their transcendental experience, the ancient *Rishis* recognized that *Mahakāla,* the timeless origin of time, is both accessible within the subjective aspect of creation, and beyond the structure of all things. It enfolds all things in its Nature. The macro and micro-worlds are integrated under laws of unified forces, as we are all aware. The existential heavenly mansions, with their planets etc. all contribute. Such are the regulating forces that guide our lives. The *Kalapurusha* concept relating the parts of the human body to the twelve *Rashis* (Figure 1.1) further expresses this in the science of *Jyotisha* astrology. In *Jyotisha,* being a Sidereal system, the *Rashis* are fixed, 30° wide, regions of the Zodiac.

In this context, *Jyotisha* astrology sets the scene to understand the possibility of *subtle* regulation of the physiology. Scientific details are discussed later under complexity biology: the physiology is regulated from *instabilities.* Over the last half century, research in complexity biology has identified instability as the universal condition for control of biological systems. It extends the study of related aspects of physiological control like internal biorhythms. These become circadian rhythms when coupled to external driving cycles; the daily cycle of light and dark driven by the sun etc. All affect regulation; depend on energy use, basal metabolic regulation etc. All such influences on biochemical molecules form Languages of Nature which *Jyotisha's Navagrahas* influence. Changing levels of amino acids are expressions of the form of Cosmic Law, in which the chemical elements constitute the 'Alphabet of Nature'.

FIGURE 1.1: Kalapurusha

The Ideal Human Body formed from the 12 *Rashis* (Jyotisha's 'Signs of the Zodiac')

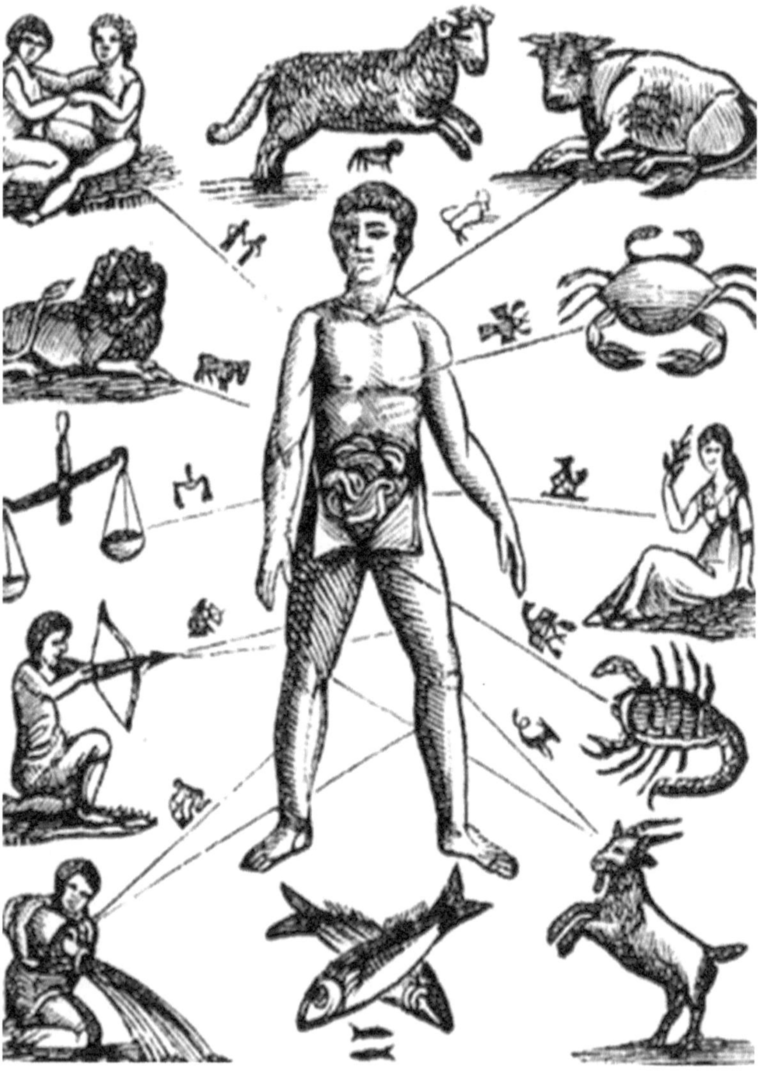

Figure 1.1 Depicts the form of the Cosmic Body of man, the *Kalapurusha,* in terms of the 12 *Rashis*.

When through experience of *Jyotisha* astrology or other Vedic sciences, higher understanding of life dawns, our minds lose their sense of privacy. Time and place significant to lower consciousness affects us less. Finally, they no longer affect our BMR; they no longer cause stress; we become established in the field of Absolute Consciousness, *Brahman.* Energy is conserved in that process. All shortfalls are resolved, whether of insulin, glucose uptake, or oxygen intake. Such problems no longer arise. Refinement of Consciousness gives rise to higher quality *Agni.* All impurities burn off. Health is promoted. Gaining the highest knowledge is like an ideal Health Care Program. We become One with Nature. Her Cosmic Mind can then guide us through all difficulties; she starts ruling us, rather than our small mind, standing alone in self-imposed isolation. Total relaxation establishes over our body; Absolute Health becomes dominant. Such is the inner message of *Jyotisha,* in keeping with all the Vedic sciences' higher understanding, to which we return in the Epilogue.

The outer message of *Jyotisha,* concerning the influence of cosmic intelligence on all our life events, is the concern of the intervening chapters, which demonstrate a scientific means of establishing its value and validity. Its inner message supports the enlightenment of the soul. Its outer message shows how to maintain optimal functioning of Body and Mind, Health. Their combination brings fulfilment to the body-mind-soul complex.

COSMOS

GALAXY

SOLAR SYSTEM

LIFE ON EARTH

ALL LIVING CELLS
ANIMALS PLANTS FUNGI BACTERIA etc.

Figure 1.2 Cosmic Intelligency in a Nutshell: Its Diagrammatic Form

Chapter 2

OVERVIEW OF THE EXPERIMENTS STRENGTHS AND WEAKNESSES

2.1 Introduction

The biological testing of *Jyotisha* astrology predictions was carried out in four series of experiments covering three areas of microbiology and veterinary science: vaccination of small ruminants, growth of bacteria, and propagation of viruses. Details of each series of experiments and their results are given in the chapters that follow. Chapter 3 presents the experiments on vaccination of small ruminants, and the difficulties they faced; Chapter 4, the bacterial growth experiments, Chapter 5 those on virus propagation, and Chapter 6, four experiments testing solar eclipse influences. In all cases, the biological processes exhibit huge variability, which is poorly understood. The variability is taken to represent experimental noise, but it is not only due to noise. Current theory is inadequate; sources of the variance need to be identified. That would improve understanding of the biological processes involved, even of biology itself.

Similar considerations apply to the second, third and fourth series of experiments, growth of pathogenic bacteria for bacterial vaccines for the second series, and propagation of viruses for viral vaccines for the third and fourth series of experiments. All the processes exhibit highly variable output, no matter what microbiological protocols are adopted. Microbiology teachers inform their students of the average growth to be expected from such processes, but not of the extreme variability that they may expect; they simply do not understand it.

The vaccinations were performed on two breeds of sheep and one breed of goats; those on the second breed of sheep were done nine months after the first, adding another element, *Rahukala*. Bacterial growth was assessed at a sequence of selected starting times on several closely spaced days, eight in the first experiment, seven in the second. Virus propagation was assessed starting at different times of day in six experiments. The first virus experiment was performed on four days, while the other five were performed on single days, three of which were selected because they were solar eclipses, the two in 2012, and the first in 2013. These three solar eclipse experiments could be compared, because the same virus and system of virus propagation was employed as in the first virus experiment. The other two virus experiments were performed on chicken viruses by two companies making avian vaccines, at the invitation of the owners.

The experiments on days of solar eclipses require special comment. The 3 solar eclipses passed nowhere near Bangalore, not even India. However, the attitude of *Jyotisha* to eclipses makes it clear that effects may be expected globally. *Jyotisha* considers the sun a very important *graha*. Later systems of Hindu devotional practice consider it worthy of worship. When the sun is eclipsed and the shadow is touching the earth anywhere, the debilitating effect is felt by all.

Jyotisha considers that, at such times, the entire structure of the subtle energies of the *grahas* has been greatly weakened. They are poor times for starting any undertaking. One should wait for at least three hours after the moon's shadow has left earth's surface; better until next day. It was therefore natural to hypothesize that even in a process as simple as virus propagation, outcomes would be systematically altered during the time of the eclipse, no matter from where the eclipse was visible. On days when solar eclipses were making their transit across the surface of the Earth, virus propagation was therefore started at five to eight selected *Muhurthas,* always including both 'eclipse times' when the sun's shadow was touching the earth, and 'non-eclipse times', either before or after that time period.

Regarding the technicalities of the experiments, their design and implementation: all the protocols were standard protocols supervised by senior professional scientists, and were carried out either by themselves, or skilled professional technicians. The initial series of experiments on vaccination, being the first, were a little tentative. They were also hard to repeat owing to restrictions on visitors to most state farms, so vaccination was only used in 2007-2008 and not attempted again. The vaccine production experiments were much easier to plan and implement, thanks to the enthusiastic support of Bangalore Veterinary College's vaccine institute. They resulted in much more robust results with definite, and in the end, definitive interpretations.

The overall summary in Chapter 8 shows how consistent the results of the experiments were. It makes the story of how the experiments unfolded worth following in detail. They were a revelation to all involved. Each succeeding experiment had our hearts in our mouths, the first solar eclipse experiment, especially. But as success followed success, we were all left with a feeling of wonder, almost dizzy that we had not met with data refuting the conjectured result of each experiment. Realizing that each was consistent with the previous experiments, and that sizes of effects observed were consistent, was amazing. Even the solar eclipses mutually agreed in detail: smaller effects were observed during an annular eclipse than a total eclipse.

Was it just luck? The accumulated results strongly suggested not. The implication was that genuine, systematic effects were at work. That led to our seeking an underlying theory in terms of physical and biological sciences, an exposition of which may be found in Chapter 7.

2.2 Strengths and Weaknesses of the Experiments

Strengths: The experiments' strengths were as follows: (1) They were carried out by top-level professionals. (2) Their location was the State Veterinary Biological Institute in the State of Karnataka, South India, a state with a very high reputation in the Education and Research sectors. (3) They received guidance from authorities in the field, all of whom were scientists of Indian Government rank, S1, the highest grade. (4) They were performed as part of ongoing professional programs of vaccine production, so the usual high professional standards were maintained. (5) The technicians who performed the experiments and made the measurements were blind to details of the research hypotheses. (6) The experiments were unbiased. (7) They were designed so data from different experiments could be combined. On a practical level: (8) The results attained ultra-high statistical significance; (9) they identified new research variables; and (10) they established a new field of microbiology research.

Weaknesses: Most of the studies should be considered pilot studies, with experimental designs testing hypotheses from *Jyotisha* for the first time. While the microbiological growth protocols were standard, stated in sources like the reference manuals of Merck corporation and OIE, no reference materials were available to help design their *Jyotisha* aspects. The latter were drawn up intuitively by the first author, later informed by progressively increasing experience. Discussions between the authors and IAH&VB Director, Dr Renuka Prasad, led to improved experimental designs, and results with correspondingly higher levels of statistical significance.

The experiments are open to the following criticisms. (1) As studies of *Jyotisha,* they were carried out for the first time. Strictly speaking, they are pilot studies. (2) Nothing like the Merck manual was available to assist in designing their *Jyotisha* aspects. (3) Everything started from scratch, with experimental designs improving from experience as the experiments progressed. (4) All were based on statements from the ancient science of *Jyotisha* interpreted in a novel fashion, as scientific conjectures, specifically for the purpose of these new experiments.

Decoding metaphysical concepts is always challenging. Bridging the gap between ancient theory and modern empirical methods should be done with caution. Sections concerning the nature of time present an interpretation of the underlying philosophy of *Jyotisha,* somewhat independent of the experiments. It is best considered purely phenomenologically.

2.3 Further Considerations

Many experiments in medicine and medical biology require ethical considerations, particularly when performed on humans or animals. None of the experiments performed on *Jyotisha* were in this category. Most were on bacteria and viruses; the former using scientifically known laboratory versions of the bacteria; those on viruses used specific cell lines and chicken's eggs.

In the first series of experiments on immune response to vaccination in small ruminants, experimental protocols consisted of standard vaccinations required, and standard monitoring of effectiveness: measurements of immune response in vaccinated animals, and small control groups. All farm animals undergo routine vaccinations to keep them free of disease, and to maintain higher levels of health. Otherwise flocks can be devastated by epidemics. Not to vaccinate them would be unethical. All the vaccinations were standard and ethically accepted. Monitoring immune response is routine scientific work, carried out constantly.

Chapter 3

VACCINATION EXPERIMENTS

3.1 Introduction

The vaccination experiments constituted the original research proposal of the first author. The plan was to carry them out on a farm belonging to the state veterinary program close to the city of Bangalore. The time was selected when the highly auspicious *Graha, Guru* (Jupiter), was very strong, placed near the beginning of his 'own house' *Dhanu* (Sagittarius). The next rising sign is *Makara* (Capricorn), whose Lord, *Sani* (Saturn), is said to cause difficulties and delays. By vaccinating in both time-slots, strongly contrasting results could be hypothesized.

The animals chosen were sheep and goats, 'small ruminants' in the language of veterinary science. The experiments were planned over 90 days. Blood samples were taken at the start, after three weeks, and after three months. However, a severe storm, some six weeks into the experiment killed many of the sheep, reducing the data. A second experiment was carried out nine months later, vaccinating a different breed of sheep. The first experiment is described in section 3.2, and the second, smaller experiment, in section 3.3. The sheep deaths proved a blessing in disguise, because they led to a second, highly inauspicious *Jyotisha* condition, known as *Rahukala*, being tested. The spectacular results of this are given in section 3.4.

Table 3.1 Design of the Small Ruminant Vaccination Experiments

Table 3.1a Experimental Design: Sheep PPR Vaccination 2007.12.02					
Breed & Age	**Groups**	**Vaccinated Time Slot**	**Number of Sheep**	**Time of Vaccination**	**Serum Samples Collected**
Ram x Deccani 7-8 mos old	Group1	'Auspicious' Time *Dhanu*	21	7.52am 9.40am	Days 0 and 21
	Group 2	Inauspicious Time *Makara*	20	9.40 am 10.40am	Days 0 and 21
	Group 3	No Vaccination Controls	12	N/A	Days 0 and 21

Table 3.1b Experimental Design: Goats PPR Vaccination 2007.12.02					
Breed & Age	**Groups**	**Vaccinated Time Slot**	**Number of Goats**	**Time of Vaccination**	**Serum Samples Collected**
Osmanabadi 7-8 mos old	Group1	'Auspicious' Time *Dhanu*	20		7.52am 9.40am
	Group 2	'Inauspicious' Time *Makara*	20	9.40 am 10.40am	Days 0 and 21
	Group 3	No Vaccination Controls	6	N/A	Days 0 and 21

3.2 The First Vaccination Experiment

Setting and Design: Chellekere farm, a State Government farm in the Chitradurga District of Karnataka, was co-opted for the experiment, as sheep and goats were both available. The design of the experiment was to vaccinate two groups of twenty animals under two different Lagnas, *Dhanu* and *Makara*, compared to unvaccinated control groups of six animals. See Table 3.1.

The experiment started on 2nd December, 2007, using the two rising signs. Things turned out differently from intended for the sheep. The *Dhanu* group had 21 animals (a counting error!), and *two* control groups of 6 were included, 53 in total. Goats numbered 46 as intended.

The measurements from the usual method of assessment of the sheep and goats are given in Table 3.2 (goats first). Considering the raw data of c-Elisa values themselves constitutes a more accurate quantitative method of assessment and is presented next.

Table 3.2 Numbers of Vaccination Successes and Failures

Goats	Total	Yes (Success) (Good Response)	No (Failure) (Smaller Response)	p Values
Group-1 (*Dhanu*)	20	**12**	**8**	**FE** 2-tailed 0.2049
Group-2 (*Makara*)	20	7	**13**	**FE** 1-tailed 0.1025
Group-3 (Control)	6	0	6	
Sheep				
Group-1 (*Dhanu*)	20	**13**	**8**	**FE** 2-tailed 0.1215
Group-2 (*Makara*)	20	7	**13**	**FE** 1-tailed 0.0789
Group-3 (Control)	12	0	12	

What was gratifying about the results of these two experiments was that they were completely consistent with each other. Both made it seem obvious that the vaccination under the first condition induced consistently better immune response, about 60% success for the first groups vaccinated under auspicious *Dhanu* (*Jyotisha* Sagittarius), but only 35% when inauspicious *Makara* (*Jyotisha* Capricorn) was the rising sign. Agreement with prediction was excellent. Figures 3.1a and 3.1b set the results out more visually in Bar Graphs.

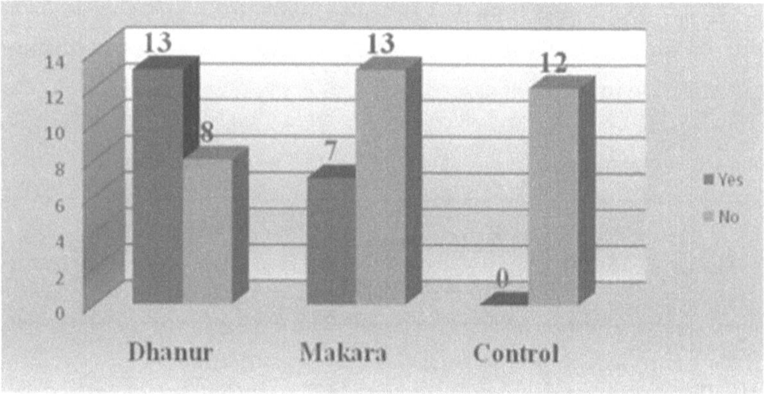

Figure 3.1a Sheep Immune Response to PPR Vaccination

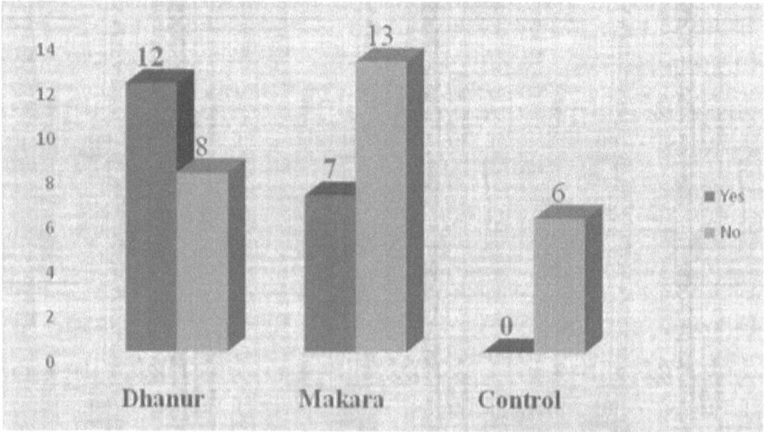

Figure 3.1b Goats Immune Response to PPR Vaccination

Because of the small numbers, the single extra sheep made a big difference to the p values measured according to Fisher's Exact test. All looks neat and clean; cut and dried, particularly when presented as bar graphs, in Figures 3.1a and 3.1b. These mutually consistent results make the experiment look spectacularly successful. But when a hard look is taken at the statistics, the all-important consideration in any scientific experiment, much is seen to be lacking. Data were taken under a distinct hypothesis, so the one-tailed probability value could be used, but in neither case could the experiment be considered conclusive. One way around this is to combine both groups of animals. Being different species means that they may not be strictly comparable; nevertheless, Table 3.2b presents combined results, which appear much more promising than those in Table 3.2.

Table 3.2b Number of Vaccination Successes and Failures: Sheep & Goats combined

Sheep+Goats	Total	Yes (Success) (Good Response)	No (Failure) (Smaller Response)	p Values
Group-1 (*Dhanu*)	41	25	16	FE 2-tailed 0.0268
Group-2 (*Makara*)	40	14	26	FE 1-tailed 0.0168
Group-3 (Control)	18	0	18	

3.3 The Second Vaccination Experiment

While the results seemed promising, they were not scientifically conclusive. They could not establish the validity of the *Jyotisha* predictions beyond reasonable doubt. More data were therefore taken on another farm in September 2008, when Guru was still well placed in its own sign, *Dhanu*, and similar astrological conditions could be obtained. The farm chosen, Dhangur, in Mandya District, close to Bangalore, breeds a different variety of sheep, Bannur.

The experimental design, set out in Table 3.3, was similar to the first experiment. Numbers were smaller, only 34 sheep in all. This time, results came out strongly in favour of *Dhanu*, as shown in Table 3.4. The effect of the *Makara* rising sign was to reduce the vaccination uptake drastically, far more than in the first experiment. The statistical significance of experiment two was better, but because the numbers were smaller, the statistics had less 'power'. They were more likely to have arisen by chance, and were therefore less conclusive.

Table 3.3 Design of the Second Sheep Vaccination Experiment

Experimental Design: Sheep PPR Vaccination 2008.09.19					
Breed & Age	**Groups**	**Vaccinated Time Slot**	**Number of Sheep**	**Time of Vaccination**	**Serum Samples Collected**
Bannur 7-8mos old	Group1	'Auspicious' Time *Dhanu*	13	12.45 am 1.01 pm	Days 0 and 21
	Group 2	'Inauspicious' Time *Makara*	10	3.03 pm 3.19 pm	Days 0 and 21
	Group 3	No Vaccination Controls	11	N/A	Days 0 and 21

The reason for the good statistical significance is that the small number of successful vaccinations under the rising sign Makara, only 2 out of 13, less than 16%, makes a huge difference to the statistics. But the small numbers reduce the reliability of the result. It really could just be chance. Strictly speaking the new data should be presented on its own, but as before, we shall combine it. Combining the figures for the two kinds of sheep gives the results in Table 3.5a.

Table 3.4 Numbers of Vaccination Successes and Failures: Bannur Sheep

Sheep	Total	Yes (Success) (Good Response)	No (Failure) (Smaller Response)	p Values
Group-1 (*Dhanu*)	10	6	4	FE 2-tailed 0.0393 FE 1-tailed 0.0367
Group-2 (*Makara*)	13	2	11	
Group-3 (Control)	11	0	11	

Table 3.5a Numbers of Vaccination Successes and Failures: All Sheep

Sheep	Total	Yes (Success) (Good Response)	No (Failure) (Poor Response)	p Values
Group-1 (*Dhanu*)	31	19	12	FE 2-tailed 0.0111 FE 1-tailed 0.0061
Group-2 (*Makara*)	33	9	24	
Group-3 (Control)	23	0	23	

These figures, for the two breeds of sheep taken together look good. A **p** value of 0.0061, about one chance in 160 of the figures occurring by chance, is satisfactory. We can try to improve the results further by combining figures for all the animals in the two experiments. Table 3.5b presents those numbers, which begin to look really impressive.

Table 3.5b Numbers of Vaccination Successes and Failures: All Sheep & Goats

Sheep & Goats	Total	Yes (Success) (Good Response)	No (Failure) (Poor Response)	p Values
Group-1 (*Dhanu*)	51	**31**	**20**	**FE** 2-tailed 0.0029
Group-2 (*Makara*)	53	**16**	**37**	**FE** 1-tailed 0.0019
Group-3 (Control)	29	**0**	**29**	

Although the scientific validity of combining all the animals together in this way might be questionable, the figures now look excellent. The bar graph Figure 7.2 makes the point strongly from a pictorial perspective. The promise of these combined results led to the experiments described in the next three chapters, Chapters 4 to 6.

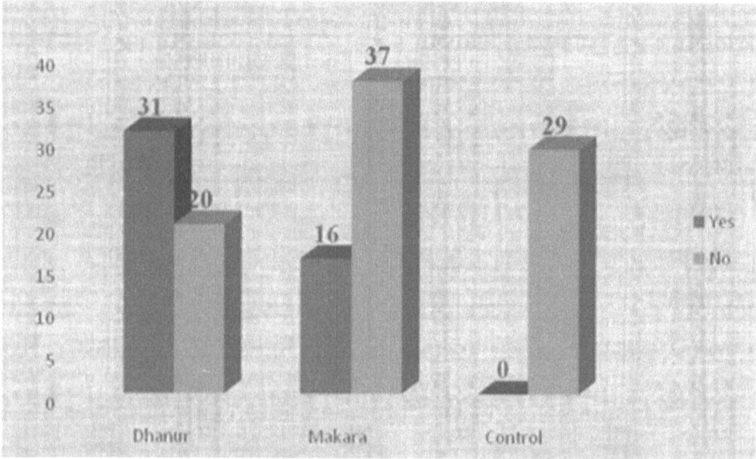

Figure 3.2 PPR Vaccination Response: All Sheep and Goats

Here, the percent success under Dhanu Lagna (60.8%) is about twice that under Makara Lagna (30.2%); the two starting times have led to very different results, across three breeds of small ruminant, two sheep and one goat.

3.4 The *Rahukala* Experiments

During the second vaccination experiment, opportunity was taken to test immune response of sheep vaccinated during a highly inauspicious time occurring every day, *Rahukala.* This is a time-period equal to 1/8th the length of the daylight hours, which occurs in a different time-slot on each day of the week. As we shall see, results of the new experiments were very striking: *none* of the animals vaccinated at those times achieved a successful immune response. The influence was far more inauspicious than *Makara Lagna,* as hypothesized. This new kind of experimental data was only taken because of the storm that interfered with the first experiment.

While the settings and methods for the *Rahukala* experiments remained the same, timings were slightly different. Times, dates and places are set out in Table 3.6, while results are presented in Table 3.7. The *Rahukala* experiments incorporated two kinds of control group: vaccinated controls (sheep of the same breed); and unvaccinated controls (also sheep of the same breed).

Table 3.6 Design of Rahukala Sheep Vaccination Experiments

Experimental Design: Sheep PPR Vaccination in *Rahukala* 2008.09.19-20					
Farm & Breed	**Groups**	**Date**	**Numbers of Sheep**	**Vaccinated Time Slot**	**Serum Samples Collected**
Chellekere Ram x Deccani	Group1	19th September 2008	12	*Rahukala* V Inauspicious	Days 0 and 21
	Group 2	19th September 2008	12	Controls	Days 0 and 21
Dhangur Bannur	Group 3	20th September 2008	13	*Rahukala* V Inauspicious	Days 0 and 21

In Chellekere Farm, since the Rahukala vaccinations were performed on different dates from the first experiment at Chellekere, serum was taken from a new control group of 12 animals. The results, set out in Table 3.7a yielded excellent statistics, which have been presented when calculated two ways, Fisher's Exact (FE) test, and the Binomial Test.

Table 3.7a Immune Response for Start-Times in *Rahukala,* Chellekere Farm

Sheep	Total	Yes (Success) (Good Response)	No (Failure) (Poor Response)	p Values
Group1 (*Rahukala*)	12	0	12	**Contingency Table**
Group-2 (Vaccinated)	41	20	21	FE2-tailed 0.0017
Group-3 (Control)	12	0	12	FE1-tailed 0.0013 **Binomial Test** 3.26×10^{-4} = 0.0003

At Dhangur Farm, serum had been taken from unvaccinated controls the previous day (Table 3.3), so no new control group of unvaccinated animals was tested. Immune response for *Rahukala* start times at Dhangur Farm, together with controls, is given in Table 3.7b.

Table 3.7b Immune Response for Start-Times in Rahukala, Dhangur Farm

Sheep	Total	Yes (Success) (Good Response)	No (Failure) (Poor Response)	p Values
Group1 (*Rahukala*)	13	0	13	**Contingency Table**
Group-2 (Vaccinated)	23	8	15	FE2-tailed 0.0820
Group-3 (Control)	11	0	11	FE1-tailed 0.0445 **Binomial Test** 3.86×10^{-3} = 0.0039

Combined results for both sets of *Rahukala* data are presented in Table 3.7c. Statistics are very significant. *Rahukala* has a very deleterious effect on immune response, as hypothesized.

Table 3.7c Immune Response for
Start-Times in Rahukala, Chellekere and Dhangur

Sheep	Total	Yes (Success) (Good Response)	No (Failure) (Poor Response)	p Values
Group1 (*Rahukala*)	25	**0**	**25**	**Contingency Table**
Group-2 (Vaccinated)	72	**28**	**36**	**FE**2-tailed 0.00003
Group-3 (Control)	23	**0**	**11**	**FE**1-tailed 0.00002 **Binomial Test** 5.6×10^{-7} 0.00000056

3.5 Conclusions

The above results show that the experiments lent strong support to both scientific conjectures tested. *Jyotisha* achieved qualitatively correct prediction of outcome. Comparison of supposed 'auspicious' starting times with supposed 'inauspicious' ones supported *Jyotisha* on their properties. Also, the 'highly inauspicious time', *Rahukala,* exerted even greater negative influence on vaccination outcomes than the mildly inauspicious time, *Makara Lagna.*

Overall, comparisons of immune response to vaccination under *Dhanu* and *Makara Lagnas* refuted the null hypothesis of no difference with excellent statistical significance in Table 3.5b. Experiments comparing vaccination under *Rahukala* and non-

Rahukala times for sheep of two breeds, similarly yielded excellent statistical significance, Contingency Table **p** = 0.00003, or **p** = 5.66 x 10^{-7} for the binomial test. Conclusions drawn from the experiments seem irrefutable.

Both combined sets of results (Table 3.5b and Table 3.7c) strongly support the study's experimental hypotheses:

1. Choice of *starting time Muhurtha* can influence outcomes of biological processes.
2. Vedic concepts of '*auspicious*' and '*inauspicious*' times possess scientific meaning: *auspicious* starting times improve vaccination uptake; *inauspicious* times decrease it.
3. *Jyotisha* astrology can make valid predictions concerning purely biological processes.

It is therefore reasonable to conclude that:

(a) The experiments strongly imply that these concepts apply to vaccination of small ruminants.

(b) Vaccination programs should take this into account, if necessary after further testing.

(c) The idea that starting time influences immune response requires further exploration, especially on humans, so that times of severely limited immune response can be avoided, and greater efficiency of vaccination achieved, both for individual vaccination, and for commercial programs of vaccination.

Chapter 4

BACTERIAL VACCINE PRODUCTION

4.1 Introduction

Following the success of the first virus vaccine production experiment described in the next chapter, it was decided to investigate possible *Muhurtha* starting time experiments on growth of bacterial vaccines, since these require simpler assessment methods than for viruses. Also, the growth protocol is simpler than for viruses, as only a single method of growth is needed (the first virus experiment used two alternatives). Rather than having only two times on the same day, the experiments had five starting times per day, and continued for several days. These improvements in experimental design helped the data produce more decisive statistics.

4.2 The Protocols and Methods

As related in Chapter 2, two series of experiments were performed by making observations on production runs of bacterial vaccines, Black Quarter (*C. Chauvoie*) vaccine, and Hemorrhagic Septicemia (*P. Multocida*) vaccine. Both experiments selected five different starting times for their production runs, including times that tradition deemed auspicious and inauspicious. The first experiment on *C. Chauvoie* vaccine production runs was conducted on 8 days between 12th October and 28th October, 2011. Growth time for each batch was 48 hours, following which growth was stopped. The second experiment observing *P. Multocida* vaccine production was conducted over 7 days in February 2012.

All the production runs were conducted according to standard scientific protocols laid out in the Merck reference text, in which IAH&VB staff were highly experienced and expert. The experiments yielded data on 40 BQ vaccine production runs, and 35 for HS vaccine.

4.3 Black Quarter Vaccine Production

For the BQ vaccine production runs, the experimental hypotheses were that *Graha Guru* would increase production, while *Rahu* would decrease it. Four different variables were measured. Data was obtained on: weight of vaccine produced, the 'Cell Mass Index' (CMI), the ability of the solution to scatter light, its 'Nephlometric Turbidity' (NTU), its ability to block light, or 'Opacity', and spore formation quality level and amount – 'Sporulation Quality'.

Data for each variable can be presented in 5 x 8 tables. One example, sporulation quality, is given in Table 4.1, since it is easy to read. Scan the Table and note the obvious pattern of rows and columns where 3's representing high quality dominate. The pattern follows the primary predictions, that times B and C when *Guru*, Jupiter, governed the rising sign at the starting time would yield best results; when *Rahu's* influence was strong, time E, they would be weakest. The data showed unexpected secondary effects: the second half of the *Guru* starting time was consistently less productive than the first half; and on certain days production was stronger than others. Those days turned out to be the ones on which the Moon was particularly strong. Evidently, the moon was also affecting the growth rates of the *C. Chauvoie* bacteria. This led to a new hypothesis for the HS experiment, which partly clarified how it was doing so.

The all-important statistical tests gave excellent results: the first, overall, level of testing called 'ANOVAs' established that the second level, called '**t**' tests' was fully justified. The **t** tests showed that the data sets contained highly unlikely patterns, with particular days, and particular starting times yielding much higher vaccine production. In both cases certain datasets yielded probabilities '**p**' of occurring by chance less than one in a million – rather like the odds on a lame horse winning a steeplechase! The pattern of **3**'s in Table 4.1 can only occur with a chance of about one in 200 million – $p = 0.5 \times 10^{-8}$. The idea that an unlikely chance pattern of events conspired to produce the results can confidently be dismissed.

Table 4.1 Vaccine Production for Black Quarter Sheep Disease

TABLE 4.1 Sporulation Quality					
DATES	A	B	C	D	E
12.10.11	1	3	2	1	1
13.10.11	3	3	3	3	2
17.10.11	1	3	2	2	1
18.10.11	2	3	2	2	2
21.10.11	2	3	2	2	3
22.10.11	2	3	2	1	1
26.10.11	1	3	2	1	1
28.10.11	1	3	2	2	1

Explanation: The first bacterial growth experiment observed standard runs of Black Quarter vaccine production, using methods following the guidelines stated in the 2012 Merck Corporation Veterinary Manual. 5 different starting times were used, on 8 days between 12th October and 28th October, 2011. Growth time for batches was 48 hrs. Data were obtained on four variables: cell mass index, nephlometric turbidity, opacity, and sporulation quality. Table 4.1 presents only the last, on sporulation quality.

Table 4.1 Caption: Table 4.1 presents the dataset on Sporulation Quality of *C. Chauvoie* after 48 hours vaccine production runs at five different times on the eight days named between 12th and 28th October 2011.

Note again: Table 4.1 shows that specific times of the day when Jupiter was strong, columns B and C, yielded highest values, and one time, column E when *Rahu* exerted a strong influence, yielded lower values, as had been predicted. Three ***days*** (the 13th, 18th, and 21st October) unexpectedly yielded higher average values than the other five. When checked, those days turned out to be days on which *Chandra*, the moon, was strong. The data table thus shows two consistent effects that had not been hypothesized. First, a strong moon can measurably enhance bacterial growth; second, it can neutralize the negative effect of *Rahu* (Col. E). All four data sets concurred on these points. These observations about *Chandra* are of intrinsic interest to *Jyotisha* astrology itself, but needed confirmation in further experiments. They were therefore included in the experimental hypotheses to be tested in the second bacterial growth experiment.

ANOVA tests yielded significant p values; t tests were conducted on the NTU data, for which the **p** values for comparisons of columns AB, AC and BC reached the required threshold. The combined product of these yielded an overall **p** of $\mathbf{5.1 \times 10^{-9}}$, five parts in a billion, about the same as the pattern of 3's in Table 4.1. The reason for citing this is explained in Chapter 8.

4.4 Hemorrhagic Septicemia Vaccine Production

Like the first bacterial growth experiment, the second also observed vaccine production runs, this time of Hemorrhagic Septicemia (HS) vaccine. Again, the experimental protocol was that for HS vaccine production given in the Merck Manual. Being aerobic rather than anaerobic, sporulation does not take place for *P. Multocida* bacteria. So, this time, only Cell Mass Index and Turbidity were measured. The two datasets, CMI and NTU, are displayed in Table 4.2.

Table 4.2 Hemorrhagic Septicemia Vaccine Production Datasets

Table 4.2a Cell Mass Index					
DATES	A	B	C	D	E
01.02.12	1.4	1.44	1.51	1.49	1.39
02.02.12	1.34	1.41	1.48	1.41	1.37
03.02.12	1.28	1.32	1.5	1.49	1.36
04.02.12	1.33	1.41	1.49	1.46	1.30
05.02.12	1.36	1.32	1.49	1.5	1.35
06.02.12	1.31	1.41	1.48	1.47	1.30
08.02.12	1.33	1.36	1.5	1.48	1.32
F (Cols = Times) = 35.45				p <0.0001	
F (Rows = Days) = 1.67				p = 0.17 NS	
2-Factor MANOVA on both data sets combined:					

Table 4.2b NTU Data					
DATES	A	B	C	D	E
01.02.12	94	98	62	145	118
02.02.12	107	92	124	126	122
03.02.12	51	62	62	63	51
04.02.12	80	78	90	98	82
05.02.12	57	60	62	61	44
06.02.12	141	182	221	174	141
08.02.12	114	154	164	187	115
F (Cols = Times) = 2.40				p = 0.0781	
F (Rows = Days) = 29.65				p< 0.0001	
Cols p = 0.00001, Rows p = 0.0024					

Tables 4.2 Caption: These two Tables present datasets from production runs of HS vaccine at five different times on the seven dates given in the left-most columns of each Table. Cell Mass Index data in grams is given in Table 4.2a, and spectrophotometer-based nephlometric turbidity data in NTU in Table 4.2b. 2-Factor MANOVA F values for their columns and rows, and corresponding p values, are given underneath each.

Results were like those for the BQ experiment. The first, ANOVA, statistical tests, indicated strong dependence on the two factors with significant p values. However, Table 4.2a for Cell Mass Index showed a stronger dependence on times of day, i.e. variations due to *Guru* and *Rahu*, while Table 4.2b showed greater dependence on days when *Chandra*, the Moon, was strong. A method of combining the two datasets into a single table gave $\mathbf{p} = 2.4 \times 10^{-8}$.

At first, the difference between days and times dependence in the two tables was mystifying: why should the moon affect values of one variable, but not the other? Finally, an explanation was found: the CMI data depends on the total mass of the cells, whereas the NTU data depends more on the number of cells in solution. *Guru* has a 'quality' of 'weight', and helps people increase their weight. Carrying this over to cells explains *Guru's* effect of increasing CMI. *Chandra*, on the other hand, represents 'Mother'. The moon may therefore be expected to help cells divide, i.e. have offspring, and stimulate cell division earlier in the life cycle. More cells of a smaller size would increase light scattering, and therefore increase turbidity.

4.5 Comments and Conclusions

The two experiments observed consistent effects, with the influence of *Guru* and *Chandra* increasing measures of growth, and that of *Rahu* opposing it. This is opposite from the experimental results on viral vaccine production presented in the next two chapters, for easily understood reasons: *Guru* and *Chandra* basically support life, while *Rahu* opposes it.

The discovery in the first experiment on BQ vaccine production that the moon also exerts a large influence was unexpected. Scientifically, it is called a '*post-hoc* observation'. The effect of a strong moon was observed to be beneficial to bacterial growth. Reflection suggested that this agrees with the role assigned to Moon in *Jyotisha* as the 'Mother of all Life'. It therefore became an additional experimental hypothesis to test in subsequent experiments.

When the second bacterial experiment on HS vaccine production was performed some four months later in February, 2012, *Chandra*'s beneficial influence on vaccine production levels on certain days was one of the experimental hypotheses; a *scientific conjecture* to be tested. The NTU dataset from the HS experiment, Table 4.2b, supported it with good statistical significance. Finding that the experimental data for the HS vaccine production runs confirmed all the experimental hypotheses with good statistical significance was very pleasing. The previously observed influences of *Guru, Chandra* and *Rahu* repeated. This inspired the group to continue with more imaginative experiments, those on solar eclipses presented in chapter 6.

More detailed analysis of the bacterial growth data, not presented showed the residual variance after the factors Days and Times of Day had been removed were 26.5% and 47% respectively. This has strong implications for attempts to explain variances in bacterial growth rates. *Variations that correlate with external variables cannot be purely random; they must have causes related to those variables.* Experiments to identify such causes are now under way.

Chapter 5

VIRAL VACCINE PRODUCTION EXPERIMENTS

5.1 Introduction

The first virus propagation experiments for production of virus vaccines were conducted partly because of the ruining of the vaccination data caused by the storm in the winter of 2007-2008, which killed many of the sheep; that and the unwillingness of the state farms concerned to repeat the experiments in later years. Eventually, the first author and his colleagues at Bangalore Veterinary College came up with the idea of testing vaccine growth experiments. The first to be performed was one on Blue Tongue (BT) virus propagation, in August and September, 2011. It is the first to be described, in Section 5.2 below. It produced tantalisingly positive data. An effect definitely seemed to be present. The first analysis of the statistics, before a MANOVA was performed, yielded results that were good, but not conclusive. It therefore led to further vaccine production experiments being performed, the first of which was the BQ bacterial vaccine experiment described in the previous chapter.

The next virus experiment, that on the propagation of the avian Raniket virus in chicken eggs, was the result of an enthusiastic offer made to Rameshrao by a client, when he learned of the new experiments during a Jyotish consultation in September, 2011. As the owner of a vaccine production company, he was happy for his next round of vaccine production to be performed in accordance with Rameshrao's protocol of suggested starting times. That is described in Section 5.3 below.

The rest of the virus propagation experiments were performed using the BT virus vaccine production protocol, and another avian virus over the course of the following year and a half, but since they all pertained to solar eclipses, they are all described in the next Chapter.

Thus, four experiments were conducted in all on BT viral vaccine production *in vitro* by virus propagation in appropriate host cells, because it seemed to work well for testing starting time effects. One used the Raniket virus that causes fatality to chickens, employing standard propagation in 9-day old chicken embryos. The final virus propagation experiment described at the end of the next chapter was another solar eclipse experiment. It was performed by a different vaccine production company in Bangalore making Reo avian virus vaccines.

5.2 The First Blue Tongue Virus Experiment

This experiment was the first microbiological experiment on effects of *muhurtha* on microbial growth. Only two starting times were used, but since there are two ways to present the cells being used for viral infection, both were employed, meaning that there were four experimental runs to compare, on each of four days: 16 in all. Results are presented in Table 5.1.

TABLE 5.1 BT Virus Infection of BHK21 (Cell Line 13) Cells for Two Starting Times

DAY⇩ TIME ⇨	Cultivation Method	TIME A $TCID_{50}$	TIME B $TCID_{50}$	Time B value minus Time A value
		Thula Lagna	Rahukala	Rahukala - Thula Lagna
Day 1 25.08.11	Monolayer	5.76	6.31	+ 0.55
Day 1 25.08.11	Cocultivation	5.36	6.24	+ 0.88
Day 2 29.08.11	Monolayer	4.75	5.25	+ 0.50
Day 2 29.08.11	Cocultivation	4.63	4.75	+ 0.12
Day 3 02.09.11	Monolayer	5.00	6.00	+ 1.00
Day 3 02.09.11	Cocultivation	4.00	5.00	+ 1.00
Day 4 06.09.11	Monolayer	5.18	7.66	+ 2.48
Day 4 06.09.11	Cocultivation	5.00	7.24	+ 2.24
	Mean	4.96	6.06	1.10
	St Deviation	0.525	1.038	0.836
		Paired t and p Values		3.72 / 0.0074

Table 5.1 Caption: Table 5.1 presents values of Bluetongue virus concentration obtained from Viral Vaccine production runs of two types, Monolayer and Cocultivation, started during two different time slots on four days selected from 25th August, 2011 to 6th September, 2011, named in the left-most column.

The Bluetongue virus was propagated in Baby Hamster Kidney BHK21 cells according to two standard OIE protocols in which the laboratory was experienced, Cocultivation and Monolayer. The assay for virus concentration was the standard HA virus titration, in which the laboratory was also immensely experienced. The experiment compared runs started at the inauspicious time of *Rahukala*, which was hypothesized to increase virus growth, with another, more auspicious time, when the *Jyotisha* sign of Libra, *Thula*, was rising. The null hypothesis was that no differences were to be expected over the 120 hour incubation period. Inspection of the data in the table reveals that virus concentration levels at auspicious Time A were consistently less than those at the inauspicious Time B. *Rahu*'s effect was to increase virus propagation. Results in Table 5.1 are easy to analyse visually. *Rahukala* gave more virus than *Thula* Lagna in all eight cases. The chance of obtaining the hypothesized result by random processes is (1/2). For all eight to come out right, the overall probability is $(1/2)^8$, $\mathbf{p} = 0.0039$. Similarly, the '**t**' test between the two columns, yields $\mathbf{t} = 3.72$, $\mathbf{p} = 0.007$. A more sophisticated MANOVA analysis, for *days, times* and *modes of growth* yielded a far better overall value, $\mathbf{p} = 6.4 \times 10^{-6}$.

5.3 Raniket Virus Vaccine Production

This experiment was the first to be performed by an independent organisation, not associated with Bangalore Veterinary College. Normal production was assessed. At each time, 200 Bobcock chick embryos were infected in 5 groups of 40. Standard OIE procedures were used. Table 5.2 presents the data. Note that there are two maxima, one at 11.00 am and one at 1.00 pm: two consistent maxima within a two-hour period precludes conventional explanations in terms of biorhythms, where only a single maximum may be expected in a 24 hour cycle.

The data show consistent clustering of the same values in each column, as expected. According to the sceptical view, any variations in the experimental data should be distributed at random, and not associated with an external factor like time. The null hypothesis thus states that any variations in the data must be purely due to chance.

TABLE 5.2 Growth of Raniket Virus in Bobcock Embryos (78 hour Protocol)

A 10.00am		B 11.00am		C 11.20am		D 12.05pm		E 1.00pm		F 3.00pm		G 4.25pm	
Group	Titre Dilution	Group	Titre Dilution	Group	Titre Dilution	Group	Titre Dilution	Group	Titre Dilution	Group	Titre Dilution	Group	Titre Dilution
A1	**10**	B1	**11**	C1	**10**	D1	**10**	E1	**11**	F1	**10**	G1	**9**
A2	**10**	B2	**11**	C2	**10**	D2	**10**	E2	**11**	F2	**10**	G2	**9**
A3	**10**	B3	**11**	C3	**10**	D3	**10**	E3	**11**	F3	**10**	G3	**9**
A4	**10**	B4	**11**	C4	**10**	D4	**10**	E4	**11**	F4	**10**	G4	**9**
A5	**10**	B5	**11**	C5	**10**	D5	**10**	E5	**11**	F5	**10**	G5	**9**
A	**10**	**B**	**11**	**C**	**10**	**D**	**10**	**E**	**11**	**F**	**10**	**G**	**9**

Table 5.2 Caption: Batches of 200 fertilized Bobcock Chicken Eggs, A to G, were divided into five groups of forty. At the 7 times in the top line, they were infected with Raniket virus according to standard procedures. Two times, B and E, were under strong inauspicious influence, while time G was under a strong auspicious influence. Methods are contained in Appendix A4.

This statement can be tested by a statistical test known as 'Fisher's Permutation Test'. Applying this test yields a probability value, **p** = (5!10!20!/35!) x (7!/4!2!1!) where the first factor expresses the combinations of the figures for the 35 batches five at a time in columns, five 9's, ten 11's, and twenty 10's, while the second expresses the number of ways of rearranging the seven columns, with four columns of 10s, two of 11's, and the last one of 9's.

The value for **p** is close to 10^{-11}, one in ten billion, far smaller than the conventionally smallest **p** value quoted of 0.0001. We shall use that tiny, tiny, one-in-ten-billion value later, when assessing the effects of all the experiments together.

Professional reactions to the data were interesting. When a paper describing these results was submitted to a leading Indian scientific journal, the reviewers opined that the data was inadequate for publication in a top journal for three reasons. (1) The nature of the assay includes subjective judgment; (2) those performing assays were not totally blinded; and (3) the assay used should not be considered powerful, consistent or accurate enough to form the basis for a major new scientific discovery. Of these, only Point 1 had any substance.

Point (2) can be answered as follows, the technicians only knew which samples were taken at the same time, but not the hypothesis concerning the different samples. While a tendency to score samples taken at the same time in agreement with each other may have been present, there could not have been any tendency to make the 7 columns agree with predictions. The probability of the 7 columns arranging their values correctly, to agree with predictions is $(4!2!1!/7!) = (1/105)$ i.e. $\mathbf{p} < 0.01$, a respectable probability by conventional standards.

Point (3), on the other hand, is spurious. Any inherent weakness in the assay would only reduce the statistical significance of the final result, but that is excellent. If not ideal, the assay must have been good enough for the stated purpose. The data therefore establishes beyond any possible doubt the hypothesis that batches of chicken eggs infected at different starting times yield different results, and that auspicious and inauspicious tendencies were followed as predicted. Two of the reviewers' three points are therefore invalid.

5.4 Comments and Conclusions

These two experiments were highly encouraging. They came at a time when the research was in a crisis. The offer by IAH&VB Director, Dr Renukaprasad, to collaborate offered many new possibilities, and was accepted with gratitude. The fact that the data in Table 5.1 was consistent, and in agreement with the experimental hypotheses encouraged the research team greatly. The positive results stimulated great enthusiasm, and motivated the experiments that followed, bacterial, viral and avian.

Chapter 6

SOLAR EXCLIPSE EXPERIMENTS

Four experiments were performed during the two solar eclipses that occurred in 2012, and the first one in 2013. The two 2012 eclipses were monitored by Bluetongue virus experiments as in the previous chapter, while the third eclipse was monitored by both that means, and a second experiment involving another Avian Virus, the Reo Retro Virus, rather than the Raniket Virus.

6.1 The First Three Solar Eclipse Experiments

The previous experiments showed (Chapters 4 & 5) that large fractions of the variances in microbial growth processes depend on the starting time of the growth process, i.e. when the flasks were infected by the microbes, bacteria or viruses. Observed influences corresponded well to the traditional concepts of 'auspicious' and 'inauspicious' times. In *Jyotisha* astrology, the best known 'inauspicious time', is a solar eclipse; they are considered so inauspicious that people are advised not to go outside during the time of an eclipse, whether or not it is visible at the point where one is located. As long as the eclipse is touching some part of the earth, a powerful negative influence is being generated, and one counters this by resting indoors.

This led to the idea of investigating virus propagation during the time of a solar eclipse. In 2012, there were two solar eclipses. The experiments were so successful that they continued to include the first solar eclipse in 2013. In all cases the influence of eclipse and non-eclipse starting times were compared, and also that of *Rahukala,* in order to try to estimate the comparative levels of 'inauspiciousness' of the two conditions. The Bluetongue virus protocol described in Chapter 5 is simple and had performed well, so it was used in these experiments.

The First Solar Eclipse Experiment (Monday 20.05.2012): Seven starting times were selected between 2.30 am and 2.00 pm, with four separate batches of virus culture started at each time. The time slots consisted of the six rising signs from Pisces (*Meena*) to Leo (*Sinha*), i.e. Pisces, Aries, Taurus, Gemini, Cancer, and Leo. Rahukala lasted from 7.40 am to 9.10 am. To test the experimental hypothesis that different starting times would yield observably different results, a preliminary ANOVA test was performed on the columns of four values, obtained at each time. This test yielded $F = 2.52$, $p = 0.054$, strongly suggesting that an effect was present, but that more data was needed to establish a rigorous $p < 0.05$ significance for the overall data. Although this result was only marginal statistically, differences between eclipse times in the first four columns and non-eclipse times in the last three columns was assessed using a 't' test between the two blocks of data. The value obtained for **t**, 3.13, yielded (for the 26 degrees of freedom) $\mathbf{p} = 0.0043$, pointed to almost certain, 'Yes!' These results stimulated the second eclipse experiment.

The Second Solar Eclipse Experiment (Wednesday 14.11.2012): The experimental protocol for the second eclipse experiment used the same virus infection procedure, employing eight time-slots, between 1.00 am and 4.00 pm. Again, four different batches were starting during each of the eight rising signs from Leo to Pisces, i.e. Leo, Virgo, Libra, Scorpio, Sagittarius, Capricorn, Aquarius and Pisces. This time, the *Rahukala* time period fell under Aquarius. The solar eclipse occurred during the first three time-slots selected. The ANOVA yielded F = 2.90, giving p = 0.02 (df = 7/24) clearly demonstrating that effects were present. The '**t**' test between the first three, eclipse time, columns, and the last five, non-eclipse time, columns, yielded **t** = 3.81, and **p** = 0.0006 (1 chance in about 1,700) demonstrating that 'eclipse' and 'non-eclipse' starting time slots produced distinctly different influences. Interestingly, the influence of *Rahukala* in column 7 of the data seemed to be at least as strong as the eclipse – its virus production value was marginally higher than those of the first three, 'eclipse-time', columns.

Since the two experiments had been set up in precisely the same way, it was possible to combine time and perform the statistical tests on the two data sets combined. When this was done, the statistical tests were performed on all fifteen columns of data. The ANOVA yielded F = 2.68, and **p** = 0.0062 against the Null Hypothesis. The t test between eclipse times (six columns totalling 24 values) and non-eclipse times (seven columns totalling 28 values) yielded **t** = 4.49, and $p = 3 \times 10^{-5} < 0.0001$. In other words, the results merit being taken very seriously. Finally, a '**t**' test between the two sets of eclipse data, the first four columns from the first experiment, against the first three columns of the second experiment, yielded **p** = 0.026 < 0.05 The significant difference suggested the 2nd eclipse exerted a stronger effect than the first. This might have been hypothesized: the first eclipse was an annular eclipse, leaving a small circle of light surrounding the moon's silhouette on the sun, but the second eclipse was total, because the moon, being closer to the earth at that point in its orbit, obscured the face of the sun completely. In contrast, the '**t**' test between the two sets of non-eclipse times, the last three columns in the first experiment, and the last four in the second experiment was not significant, as expected, suggesting that any results were not spurious.

The Third Solar Eclipse Experiment (Friday 10.05.2013): A third experiment was performed on the first solar eclipse in 2013, occurring on 10th May. Five different starting time slots were selected between 6.30 am and 3.30 pm: the four rising signs Taurus (*Vrishabha*), Gemini (*Mithuna*), Leo (*Sinha*) and Virgo (*Kanya*), and a *Rahukala* time slot in the middle, when Cancer (*Karka*) was rising. The first three times yielded higher levels of virus production than the last two.

Combining the data sets from the three eclipses, and performing an ANOVA yielded an 'F' value, $F = 3.17$, for which **p** was 0.0003, less than one part in three thousand. The null hypothesis is clearly rejected. Comparing eclipse (32 values from eight times) and non-eclipse (36 values from nine times) data yielded $t = 4.53$, with **p** far less than 0.0001 ($df = 66$), highly significant. Solar eclipse effects cannot be doubted. The published paper describing these three experiments is contained in the appendix.

6.2 Avian Reo Virus Solar Eclipse Experiment (Also Friday 10.05.2013)

Another solar eclipse experiment was conducted during the 10th May 2013 eclipse. Differences between eclipse and non-eclipse starting times were evaluated by the immune response to inactivated Avian REO virus, the standard vaccine to protect chickens against REO virus.

Avian REO Viruses, double-stranded RNA viruses of the genus *Orthoreovirus*, are important commercially, because they can cause poultry growers considerable losses. Most REO virus infections have no serious consequences, but some produce arthritis (tenosynovitis) in birds 4–16 weeks of age, affecting production and quality of meat. Large outbreaks in flocks of commercial chickens cause severe loss of value. Vaccination is necessary. Infected birds have circulating antibodies, as demonstrated by various kinds of test.

Eight-week old COBB breed chickens were vaccinated against REO virus in batches of 30 during each of five time slots. Two time-slots were eclipse times, one was *Rahukala,* and two were non-eclipse time-slots, i.e. after the path of the eclipse had finally left the earth's surface. Blood samples were taken prior to vaccination, and 6 weeks afterwards. REO-ELISA tests were performed to measure increases in REO virus antibodies. Raw data consisted of optical density (OD) values from the c-ELISA tests. Mean increases in values for each of the batches, together with their standard deviations, were used in the data analysis.

The statistical analysis yielded remarkable results. The statutory ANOVA yielded $F = 7.08$, and $p < 0.0001$, showing that there is excellent significance in response to the question, "Is there a difference between results of experiments started at different times?" The null hypothesis of no response was categorically rejected.

The '**t**' tests yielded **t** values between the two Eclipse-Time columns and the two Non-Eclipse-Time columns, $\mathbf{t}_1 = 4.3$, $\mathbf{t}_2 = 4.5$, $\mathbf{t}_3 = 2.42$, $\mathbf{t}_4 = 3.09$, for which the **p** values were, $\mathbf{p}_1 < 0.0001$, $\mathbf{p}_2 < 0.0001$, $\mathbf{p}_3 = 0.018$, and $\mathbf{p}_4 = 0.003$ respectively. Combining these four by multiplying them together yields an overall statistic of $\mathbf{p} < 0.72 \times 10^{-12} < 10^{-12}$. As we shall see, this remarkably tiny result contributes significantly to the overall statistical significance of all the experiments taken together. Regarding the *Rahukala* measurements, data showed that it produced values distinct from eclipse or non-eclipse times. *Rahukala*'s influence differed from both.

The conclusion of the REO Virus vaccination experiment was that vaccinations performed during eclipse and non-eclipse times have distinct, different effects. *Rahukala* seemed to exert an influence intermediate between the two. Overall, the results were consistent with, and supported, the conclusions of the other three eclipse experiments.

6.3 Implications

The first three experiments combine with the fourth to provide strong support for the concepts of 'auspicious' and 'inauspicious' times, and the hypotheses that levels of virus propagation increase at times considered inauspicious and decrease at those deemed auspicious. A major strength of these four experiments was that the *first three eclipse results using BTV virus propagation were consistent with those using REO virus.*

Overall, the experiments indicate that starting times during an eclipse exert an influence on biological processes, even at locations not touched by the eclipse. None of the eclipses touched the Indian subcontinent, yet their effects were clearly observed. This implies that eclipses generate some kind of global influence on the biosphere, an idea that requires further experimental investigation. We suggest that the observations support a new form of Gaia hypothesis that the biosphere may function as a single global entity as apparently observed here. Their wider implications are that on days of solar eclipses, at least some influences on the biosphere are global, and may be negative from a healthcare perspective.

Chapter 7

A PHYSICAL THEORY OF ASTROLOGY

Combining Complexity Biology and Quantum Theory

7.1 Introduction

As we have seen, the idea that astrology may be described by a scientific theory is impossible for most scientists to conceive. Consider Quine's dichotomy, that anyone believing in astrology must reject scientific laws, because science and astrology are incompatible. Just that kind of problem appeals to the second author. Thorough study of any science, physics, chemistry or biology, leads one to see the field's weak spots, places where new possibilities lie hidden. When faced with seemingly real phenomena like *Jyotisha*, the conviction arises that behind it there lie reasons connected to already developed scientific ideas. In 1972, when discussing a new and unexplained, but well-established phenomenon in material science, Steven Weinberg remarked, "There must be a reason for that." Indeed, there was, a theory of those phenomena won Weinberg's colleague, Ken Wilson, a Nobel prize a decade later.

Experiments establishing astrological influences on micro-organisms are equally enthralling. Likewise, "There must be a reason for them." In the case of astrology, Weinberg stated that it was not worth his time and effort to pursue. His former student thought otherwise! Before considering such a radical new theory, observe a feature of all truly novel scientific theories: they usually require two separate extensions to previous scientific theories; one in each of two fields. When faced by phenomena that are clearly impossible to explain by extending a single field, two separate, seemingly unrelated extensions of two different fields are needed to find an appropriate theory. Such theories are nigh-on impossible to conceive, let alone find. Considerable luck is needed to hit on the right combination of innovations, and then show how to integrate them. Only then can otherwise inexplicable data be explained.

From science's perspective, *Jyotisha* is just one of several fields of traditional knowledge in which seemingly inexplicable phenomena occur. This chapter shows, nevertheless, how to construct a *bona fide* theory of *grahas* influence on organism functions, down to single cells. The theory requires combining new ideas in both biology and astrophysics: biology, to identify structures that can be influenced; astrophysics, to explain how *grahas* may affect them.

First, we present the new theory in outline. Readers who find scientific technicalities difficult to follow need not struggle with the main sections of this chapter. Equally, those who want to understand the technical details can start with a bird's eye view, aimed to make reading easier.

The scientific landscape that we shall traverse is not familiar. The two subfields used to construct a theory of *Jyotisha*, are *Complexity Biology* and hitherto neglected *quantum properties* of the *Navagrahas* in astrophysics. Thousands of papers in complexity biology have demonstrated that all biological functions are exceedingly delicately controlled. Their 'Loci of Control' are at *instabilities*, of a kind like those in critical phenomena for which Ken Wilson won his Nobel prize. Such phenomena are susceptible to quantum influences.

In astrophysics, planets are such large physical bodies that no one has ever proposed that, in addition to classical properties of mass, momentum, energy, temperature, and gravitational and magnetic fields, they might possess distinct quantum properties. Never has anyone had reason to consider that they might. But, as will be shown, the formation of the solar system involves processes inevitably embedding vast quantities of internal quantum coherence in each *graha*. Such quantum coherence has the power to shift balance points of biological regulation. Any physiological function may be influenced, and observable effects on its output produced. So delicately sensitive and responsive is physiological regulation at instability.

There in a nutshell, is the kernel of the new theory. *Biological regulation has unheard of sensitivity – far more delicate than any man-made control system. So delicate is that instability-based sensitivity, that quantum correlations in grahas can influence it, correlations generated when the solar system formed.*

Few scientists know the facts of complexity biology, to the extent that one Past President of London's Royal Society has been at pains to emphasize its significance. The field is now reaching maturity. Further, no one has considered that biological loci of control are so sensitive that quantum correlations can influence them. Equally, no one has explained how large quantities of quantum correlations accumulate in planetary interiors during their accretion. That idea is also new. Put together, the two combine to predict that the *Navagrahas* exert measurable influences on regulated biological processes. A theory of astrology has been born!

The next section sets the scene with examples of new theories. Subsequent ones fill in missing details, to give a full understanding of all aspects of the proposed theory – science's first attempt to offer a *bona fide* theory of astrological phenomena predicted by *Jyotisha.*

7.2 New Theories in Science

This section describes four major scientific theories that were very difficult to 'see' for the first time, and almost impossible to discover. Initial conception required outstanding power of intuition and creative cognition. They cover mathematics and physics and concern such famous figures as Archimedes, Newton and Weinberg. They date from hundreds of years B.C.E. to the final decade of the 20th century.

The most recent, celebrated example of radical new theory was the proof of Fermat's last theorem by Andrew Wiles of Princeton University. His work presents a fine example of new theory requiring two separate extensions to already existing work in the field – in Wiles's case, a field that he had already revolutionised. Wiles first proposed his proof of Fermat's last theorem in a surprise exposition at a conference. The lecture contained reams of new mathematics developed over the previous decade; an awe-inspiring performance, mathematics at its most brilliant, by a master of his field, whom only equally brilliant minds could follow.

After the lecture, a hidden flaw in the proof was pointed out by an eminent colleague. A seemingly minor assumption had not been fully established, and had been overlooked. Wiles realised that the flaw in his proof was a critical deficiency, which would require much deep thinking to explore and resolve. He announced that he would give himself a year to complete the task, and recruited a brilliant former student to work with him.

After many months work on a promising path, Wiles had to give up; all avenues had been explored and failed. He then worked for the rest of the year on another line of thinking utilizing a different set of principles. That proved equally fruitless. On almost the final day, having given up and relaxing after realising that he would finally have to admit failure, Wiles experienced a stroke of creative insight, an 'illumination'. He conceived, or 'saw', a pattern of reasoning that *would integrate his two different approaches.*

He realised that it offered a new possibility of success. When he tried it out in detail, all turned out as he had conceived. His creative imagination had come up with the solution. *Integrating the two approaches concluded the final steps of his proof.*

Integrating separate extensions of theories from different scientific fields is not easily achieved. Why should some new physics conceived in one field apply sufficiently closely to integrate with another field? But in science many great advances have been achieved by such means.

Consider Archimedes who sprang out of the public bath and ran to the King of Syracuse naked, when he realised that the law of ratios formulated in his law of levers could also be applied to densities of gold alloys used in making a crown; the pattern of his intellectual apprehension in solving a seemingly impossible problem is plain for all to see. Realising that his hand felt lighter when placed in the water in the bath, he 'saw' that he could use his law of ratios to answer the question given to him by the King: "Was the crown that the goldsmith was trying to sell him, pure gold? Or had it been alloyed with silver?"

Archimedes' genius had previously worked out two scientific theories: his law of the lever, applied to commercial scales, and the law of flotation – the upward force on a body immersed in water is equal to the weight of water displaced. Archimedes' intuition *combined his theory of the first problem, the lever and the balance, with his understanding of the second problem, flotation.* The *combination* provided the intuitive pattern needed to solve the King's question.

Solving problems in physics is a matter of 'seeing which pattern to use', either from prior knowledge gained by solving similar problems, or by conceiving a new pattern, which can be seen to fit the problem like a key in a lock.

7.3 Pairs of Integrated Advances in Revolutionary Theories in Modern Science

When he first realised that the kinematics of the moon's motion and those of an apple could be combined, Newton had an 'epiphany' like Archimedes. His insight led him to use both his laws of mechanics and his formulation of the law of gravity. The two theories applied in different realms, the first to objects found here on earth, while his proposed law of gravity applied to the sun, moon, planets and stars seen in the sky. Previously they had been thought to be unrelated to the kind of matter found here on earth; partly because of their *astrological* properties.

At that time, heavenly bodies were not thought to be mechanical objects. Both Galileo and Descartes had questioned the Church's judgment on this and suffered for doing so. The *grahas* were in a different category of perceived entities. Newton saw that *he could combine Galileo's kinematics* including the radical new concept of acceleration with *Descartes' coordinate geometry*, and that *the combination would enable him to use an inverse square law of gravity to explain Kepler's first law of elliptical planetary orbits with the sun at one focus.* Genius *integrating ideas from two or three fields* founded the mathematical physics practised today.

Similarly, in the 1860's, James Clerk Maxwell was working on electricity and magnetism, expressing their laws in terms of new mathematics: 'partial differential equations' in the four variables of space-time. Maxwell '*saw*' that, *to make the laws mutually self-consistent, he needed to reformulate one of the four laws concerned,* that of electromagnetic induction. He could then *integrate the two theories.*

Maxwell's radical, *integrating* step enabled him *to formulate a wave equation,* which predicted that *the waves would move at the speed of light* (or close to it). Accurate verification of his prediction showed that *he had achieved the integration of the previously disparate fields of electricity, magnetism and optics – the study of light.*

Likewise, Weinberg: when formulating the 'Standard Model' of elementary particle physics: Weinberg achieved *a sensational integration of two seemingly irreconcilable theories, electromagnetism and the weak force,* found in radioactivity. Unstable nuclei emit either an electron or its anti-particle, the positively charged positron, together with electrically neutral particles, 'neutrinos', in processes called 'beta decay'.

Previously, the two theories had seemed so different as to be conceptually irreconcilable, rather like electrical charges and magnets, or building a boat as opposed to making a beautiful silver-alloyed gold crown. Weinberg's genius was to pick up the idea that *the weak interaction might be due to very heavy particles with mathematical structures related to the photon.* This, he used *to propose a set of four, previously unobserved, heavy particles to integrate the two theories.* Sleight of hand in his deft mathematical imagination enabled Weinberg *to integrate and unify the two theories.*

More importantly, he made observable, 'conjectured', predictions, which could be tested by experiment and were later found true. The spirit, in which his unification of the two theories was conceived, was like Maxwell's when unifying electricity and magnetism. But Weinberg's theory is far more sophisticated.

7.4 Towards a Scientific Theory of Jyotisha I: Criticality in Complexity Biology

The above theories mark astonishing advances in physics. Two separate advances were needed to explain new connections, like the two piles from which a bridge is built. *Jyotisha* needs new ideas in astrophysics and biology, on which the bridge may be structured. Biology is in a state of flux. Oxford University's Professor Emeritus of Physiology, Denis Noble, finds regulation of genetic expression far more important than ever expected. Its consequences for variations in organism behaviour are far greater than imagined. Complexity is another field of discoveries of major importance. Could it be that these new fields of biology could contain the seeds of an explanation for the influence of starting time on growth process outcome?

The answer we propose is a tentative, 'Yes!' Complexity shows that biological regulation is quite different from anything imagined. All regulatory processes have 'Loci of Control', states where regulation is centred. The Loci of Control are *states of inherent instability*, 'critical instability', known in biology as 'criticality'. The reason is simple. Criticality maximizes sensitivity of system response to stimuli. It thus optimizes regulation. Biology has found a way to optimize matching internal processing with external demands, a competitive advantage.

Criticality is a complex condition. Maintaining it requires self-organizing power. Stresses can drive a 'locus of control' away from criticality, weakening system function. Regulation is less effective. Health is compromised. Restoring optimal function requires restoring regulation to optimal at criticality. At that natural locus of control, '***Optimal regulation is optimal health***'. That is why instability is found *universally* in biological regulation.

All the *Jyotisha* experiments required active organism regulation of processes involved. All had Loci of Control at criticality, points of physical instability. Here, dynamics are new and different. They must be, or stability would obtain. Stability is maintained by simple harmonic oscillations. Instead, a system property has become unstable; its values fluctuate wildly. System dynamics are governed by 'fluctuations'.

Critical fluctuations have completely different properties from simple harmonic oscillations. The latter form the basis of quantum phenomena, of all quantum fields, in materials and empty space. Critical point fluctuations cannot be described by quantum theory. They are something other. But one property, described next, allows them to interact at a quantum level.

A characteristic of criticality is that, like all instabilities, it possesses a high level of internal coherence, 'Critical Point Coherence'.

7.5 Towards a Scientific Theory of Jyotisha II: Internal Correlations

In stable matter, activity at each point is independent of activity at the next point, roughly speaking. Each atom oscillates with its own degrees of freedom, and although the strength of its oscillations influence those of neighbouring atoms, any correlations between them rapidly die away to zero, 'exponentially', in mathematical terms. Critical point fluctuations behave completely differently. Instead of reducing to zero with exponential rapidity, they only die away with some small power of the distance, d, close to (1/d). This means that correlations in a system at criticality are long-range. Having long range internal correlations, means that *physiological systems possess extremely high internal coherence.*

From an ordinary perspective, instability and internal coherence might seem internal weaknesses; especially because, as we shall see, they enable planets to exert hidden influences on organism regulation! In fact, this brings to bear the 'language of colours' of cosmic creative intelligence, so that access is a strength. And the means of that access, is through the extraordinary properties of the *Navagrahas* that we discuss next.

First, a cautionary note: prediction of long-range coupling between mutually coherent quantum systems so distressed

Einstein that he rejected quantum theory as a fundamental theory of physics. It did not accord with his intuition of Nature, how Her activity is structured. However, here his intuition on that count was wrong. The existence of long-range quantum correlations has been irrefutably demonstrated. The idea that two quantum systems can be correlated, despite being separated by vast, macroscopic distances, is now well accepted in physics.

Austrian Professor Anton Zeilinger of the University of Vienna is a top scientist who has studied the effects of quantum correlations in simple systems, and demonstrated their 'reality' in practical systems in physics laboratories. His formulation of 'Quantum Teleportation' made him one of the scientific community's most influential members. His work is highly respected.

Most people familiar with quantum correlations know only those between two quanta. But systems of many quanta often contain correlations between them all. Electrons in a single atom, such as Uranium with 92 electrons or Gold with 79 electrons, are described by single wave functions, a matrix with correlations of order 92 and 79 respectively. In lasers, all the photons are highly correlated. The order of the correlations may be many thousand or many million. The physics of high order correlations found in systems, like lasers (and superconductors) with large quantities of internal quantum correlations, is well understood.

In the case of the high levels of internal correlations in systems at critical instabilities, the same is true, but on a profoundly greater scale. In biological systems, critical correlations at their loci of control, make them sensitive to correlations in other systems; both quantum correlations, and critical correlations in other organisms. As in the case of correlations between pairs of quantum systems, the degree of correlation between two such systems does not change with distance. The influence, once established, is *independent of distance between the two systems.*

7.6 Towards a Scientific Theory of Jyotisha III: Internal Correlations in *Grahas*

An immediate consequence of Zeilinger's extensive experimental work is this: If macroscopic bodies in the solar system can be shown to contain high levels of quantum correlations, that would mean that they can influence critical instabilities in biological control systems by coupling to their internal critical correlations. But demonstrating that *grahas* contain high levels of quantum correlations is easy. Systems become correlated by interacting with each other. Collisions of any kind result in correlations between the colliding systems. If they continue independently, their momenta are at least partly correlated. If they coalesce, they gain internal correlations.

The birth of the solar system involves collisions of at first, tiny, and then increasingly large particles; dust, pebbles, rocks, boulders up to the size of asteroids and the moon. These continue to rain down on the earth and other planets, occasionally causing fearsome catastrophes, like the two, which almost wiped out life on earth in the last three hundred million years.

Each impact contributes to the growth of a moon, planetary body, planetoid, or planet. Two effects occur: one understood by classical physics, the other, in terms of quantum physics. On the level of classical physics, heat is generated, as is well understood. What is less appreciated, though no less true, is that, *on the quantum level,* ***internal quantum correlations are generated***.

Quantum correlations are an inevitable result of interactions between pairs of quantum systems. When two independent quanta are fired at each other in particle accelerators, their states, on a quantum level, are independent of each other. But after their interaction, they are strongly correlated because of the interaction between them. In the same way, condensation of planets by gravitational attraction, which causes the colliding bodies to coalesce, *creates internal quantum correlations.* Ultra-high levels result from the vast number of particles involved.

And what of *Rahu* and *Ketu,* the North and South Nodes of the Moon? The North Node is the point in the equatorial plane through which the moon passes from the south side of the plane to the north side; while the South Node is the opposite point in the its orbit through which she passes from the north side to the south side. Neither is a material body. How can they act like sources of correlations? The reasoning must be extended. Fortunately, that is easy to do. Both Nodes represent dynamic correlations between the relative motions of the sun, moon and earth. Since their positions are produced by *correlations* between these motions, the Nodes represent massive sources of potential correlational influence. This line of reasoning solves the problem.

7.7 Coupling the Two Kinds of Correlations: A Theory of Jyotisha Astrology

In biological systems, the order of the critical point correlations is roughly the number of atoms involved in the state – which could be several thousand. But in a planet, it could be equal to some significant fraction of the number of atomic particles that collided during its formation. The number is astronomically much higher – literally. Similarly, it is immensely more effective in influencing a biological control system located at an instability. The same is true of any star like the sun, or any of its planets. The order of its internal quantum correlations may be a not insignificant fraction of the total number of quanta that it contains.

In any system of planets orbiting a central star, the development of any event involving an instability on one planet in the system, or even events on the star itself, can be influenced by quantum correlations contained in any other planet, or by that planet's moon(s). Possibilities are immensely rich. The effects of *grahas* on instabilities controlling processes in physiological systems are just one example. Others include effect of *grahas* on tendencies in human minds.

7.8 Conclusions

Condensation during the birth of the solar system generated vast levels of quantum correlations in each *graha.* All *grahas* contain levels of quantum correlations that can influence instabilities anywhere in the solar system. Quantum theory predicts that the influences will be independent of distance to each *Graha,* as *Jyotisha* implicitly assumes. This first agreement between theory and practice is a major achievement. The theory starts well.

This new physics predicts that all *Grahas* interact in an entirely new way with each other. Gravitational effects are well known and well understood. Interactions between a planet's magnetic fields and the solar wind, producing the Van Allen Radiation Belts and the Aurora Borealis and Australis, are also well understood. The new physics predicts that each *graha*'s internal quantum correlations influence tendencies at every instability in the solar system. All sources of all new processes, hurricanes, humans etc. are influenced. *Every process growing out of an instability, or continuously regulated from one, will be subject to* ***Jyotisha*** *effects.*

Good reason to think that *Grahas* may really exert ongoing influences on processes on earth: possible cases include individual and collective human activities, and processes in every life-form on earth. All physiologies are regulated from *criticality.* All can be influenced by *grahas.* Take a look out of the window, every cell in every plant and animal that we see, all aspects of their higher regulation, are influenced by quantum coherence. Such influences are neither rare nor unusual; they constitute an integral aspect of biology, psychology, social science, and even meteorology; all such phenomena are under the influence of the *Navagrahas*. We may legitimately inquire about *Jyotisha* conditions leading to tropical storms that start from well-known, '*Butterfly Effect*' instabilities. We have not explained directional effects, deeper levels may explain them. Physicist, Liudmila Boldyreva, has derived results on 'Cavity Effects in Medicine', on which the authors commented. Directional effects in *Jyotisha* may relate to effects that she described. There is much to develop further in the new theory. It seems qualitatively promising, but it is still in its infancy, scientifically speaking.

Chapter 8

DISCUSSION AND CONCLUSIONS

8.1 General Discussion

The results of the ten experiments are summarized in Table 8.1. Eight were conducted by S1 Indian government microbiological scientists with highest training, reputation and experience at IAH&VB, one of South India's top biological institutes. The other two, on avian vaccines, were conducted by experienced commercial technicians. World-standard guidelines were followed from OIE or Merck Corporation.

In the animal vaccination experiments, two kinds of experiment assessed immune response to PPR vaccination in three breeds of small ruminant. The first kind, conducted on two occasions 9 months apart, compared two rising signs for vaccination of sheep and goats; the second compared the highly inauspicious time, *Rahukala,* with an average of ordinary times. Both kinds of experiment obtained excellent statistical significance. The reality of *Jyotisha* influences could not be disputed, nor that their qualitative effects were as hypothesized.

The second series of experiments began with assessment of virus propagation during viral vaccine production. The first tested Bluetongue (BT) sheep virus vaccine production during two different starting time slots, the inauspicious *Rahukala*, and a relatively auspicious time when the *Jyotisha* sign of *Thula* (Libra) was rising. The second experiment in that series assessed production of Raniket virus at seven different starting times, one auspicious and two especially inauspicious. The inauspicious starting times led to greater virus propagation, while the auspicious time led to smaller virus production. Statistical significance was again excellent.

The two experiments in the third series monitored growth of pathogenic bacteria, at five different starting times on several days selected from time periods of one to three weeks. In the first, production runs of *BQ* vaccine were started at five times on each of eight days, yielding 40-point data tables; in the second, production runs of HS vaccine were started at five times on each of seven days, yielding 35-point data tables. In both experiments, results of very high statistical significance were obtained, with the effects of three *Jyotisha grahas, Guru, Chandra* and *Rahu,* accounting for 50 to 78% of the observed variances in the assessed parameters.

The fourth kind of experiment observed production runs of two viral vaccines on days of solar eclipses, using sequences of five to eight rising signs. Various auspicious and inauspicious influences were also included, auspicious effects of *graha Guru,* and inauspicious *Rahukala.*

As informed observations of ongoing vaccine production processes, the experiments were zero-cost pilot experiments using standardized protocols. The supervising scientists knew them well. While their pilot study nature may seem a weakness, the strength of their statistics is striking (Table 8.1 right column). Full experiments with better test procedures may be more convincing for specialists, but those involved agreed that the results were highly significant.

TABLE 8.1 Ten Starting Time Experiments in Veterinary Microbiology

#	System	Vaccine	Dates	DF	p Value	Test	p value(s)
1.	Immune Response	PPR	02.12.2007 2 Lagnas	101	FET 2-Tail $p = 0.0029$	$t = 4.904$	$p_2 = 2 \times 10^{-6}$
2.	Immune Response	PPR	09.08.2008 Rahukala	24	FET 2-Tail $p = 3 \times 10^{-5}$	Binomial	$p = 5.66 \times 10^{-7}$
3.	**Vaccine Culture**	**BT Virus**	4 days, Aug & Sept 2011	**4 x 4**	**$p_1 = 0.0039$** **$p_2 = 0.0140$**	**Binomial Test**	**$p_1 = 0.0002$** **$p_2 = 10^{-6}$**
4.	**Vaccine Culture**	***C. Chauvoie***	8 Days, Oct2011	**5 x 8**	**$p_1 < 0.0001$** **$p_2 < 0.0001$**	**$F_R = 30.6$** **$F_C = 9.40$**	**$p_t <<< 10^{-8}$ (Overall)**
5.	Vaccine Culture	Raniket Virus	18.11.2011	5 x 7	$p < 10^{-11}$	Inter Column	0.24×10^{-12} (Overall)
6.	Vaccine Culture	*P. Multocida*	7 Days, Feb., 2012	5 x 7	$p_1 < 0.0001$ $p_2 = 0.0010$	$F_R = 9.83$ $F_C = 4.36$	$p_t < 10^{-7}$

#	System	Vaccine	Dates	DF	p Value	Test	p value(s)
7-9.	**Vaccine Culture**	**BT Virus Eclipses 1-3**	**20.05.2012 14.11.2012 10.05.2013**	**4 x 7 4 x 8 4 x 5**	$P_1 = 0.0538$ $P_2 = 0.0020$ $P_3 = 0.0026$ $P_{123} = 0.0003$	$F_R = 11.13$ $F_C = 11.75$	$P_R = 0.0002$ $P_C = 0.0002$ $P_T = 4x10^{-8}$
10.	Immune Response	Reo Virus Eclipse 3	10.05.2013	5 x 30	$P_1 < 0.0001$ $P_2 < 0.0001$ $P_3 = 0.018$ $P_4 = 0.003$	t = 3.81	$P_T < 10^{-12}$
Overall Result		**Using Bayesian Statistics to Combine all Eight p values**					$p = 10^{-65}$

Table 8.1 Caption: Table 8.1 presents overall statistics, including 't' & p values, for the ten experiments testing hypotheses of Jyotisha astrology Muhurtha starting time-slot predictions for processes in veterinary microbiology. The final line assesses the Null Hypothesis that, 'Jyotisha cannot make accurate statements in microbiology'

8.2 The Scientific Perspective

Scientifically, testing null hypotheses was the main aim of the experiments. In a new field of investigation, the correct scientific question is, "Does a phenomenon exist?" Precisely quantifying it by more accurate methods of measurement is the *second* stage. Refuting null hypotheses is the correct first goal. Experimental science treats both experimental hypotheses and null hypotheses, as scientific 'conjectures' to be tested. Proposed experiments are designed to refute one or the other with a reasonable degree of statistical significance.

The experiments identified a series of related effects. First, influence of starting times on outcome of microbiological processes is clearly demonstrated to good statistical significance in all the data sets. For experiments 7 to 9 on solar eclipses, combining improved the statistical results, because the three data sets were mutually consistent, supporting each other, and amplifying the statistical significance. In all cases, statistically significant refutations of the null hypothesis obtained. Some data sets yielded two significant **p** values after 2-Factor MANOVAS were performed. In experiments 5 and 10, on Raniket and Reo Virus propagation, statistics refuting the null hypothesis were astoundingly high; the result of fortuitous experimental design.

8.3 Overall Significance of the Experiments

In fields where many experiments are conducted to continue testing the same experimental hypothesis, results of many experiments are combined in 'systematic reviews' using a method called meta-analysis to evaluate their overall statistical significance. The method obtains much higher degrees of certainty that null hypotheses are wrong, and experimental hypotheses right.

In Table 8.1, results of experiments 7 to 9 have already been combined. The other experiments were of different kinds; meta-analysis is inappropriate. Instead, 'Bayesian Statistics' can be used to successively combine **p** values from each experiment into an overall **p** value, testing the overall *null* hypothesis: '***Jyotisha*** astrology cannot make accurate predictions.'

This statement presents the skeptics' scientific position. It exposes its weakness. No experiment should yield significant results. Any experiment doing so threatens their world view. Bayesian statistics' procedures can combine results of all experiments, no matter their **p** values; even experiments not yielding statistically significant results by themselves can be integrated into the overall result using its methods; **p** values over 0.05 can be included.

For the experiments described above, their tiny **p** values allow Bayesian statistics to combine them by simply multiplying the eight overall probabilities in Table 8.1's final column. As shown in the bottom row, this yields an overall **p** Value for the whole table. Strictly speaking each **p** value should be combined one at a time, starting from an initial value of **p**. What should that initial value be? The philosophy of empirical science is quite clear on the matter: *scientists must always refrain from taking sides about the null hypothesis.* They should start from an entirely detached view of it, and allow the experiments to determine the result, irrespective of initial prejudices on the matter.

Sometimes scientists say: "I won't believe results of any experiment involving statistics". But that attitude is opposed to empirical science. Errors must be estimated in every experiment so that: (1) Sources of error can be identified and hopefully removed by improved experimental protocols; and (2) the minimized errors in the final experiment can be accurately estimated. Then the statistical significance by which the null hypothesis was finally refuted can be given. *Because experimental errors must be estimated and kept in control, statistics must be employed* if only to see that they are being kept in check. The 20th century developed immense theories of statistical methods. Science holds that: *without statistics, empirical work is meaningless.*

Empirical science rests entirely on experimental testing of scientific predictions considered as 'refutable conjectures'. The validity of such conjectures depends on their ability to withstand attempts to refute them. Statistical methods estimate their validity, culminating in Bayesian analysis of all experiments, starting from an initial value of **p** representing zero experimental knowledge, without prejudice. This 'detached perspective' is given by $\mathbf{p} = \frac{1}{2}$.

Sceptics should accept that, if their beliefs and preconceptions really are true, well-designed scientific experiments will prove them right. But equally, if those preconceptions are wrong, the experiments will arrive at *the empirically correct statement with the degree of statistical certainty allowed by the power of the experimental designs employed.* That is empirical science. Of course, whether one accepts empirical methods of testing ideas is a matter of personal choice up to each of us to make. If that is uncomfortable for one's intellect, so be it.

What do the results tabulated in Table 8.1 tell us, empirically? Clearly that the null hypotheses were consistently ruled out with high degrees of certainty. The probability that the overall null hypothesis representing the sceptic position is correct is reduced by each experiment, from 2×10^{-6} after line 1 to 1.13×10^{-12} after line 2 to 1.13×10^{-18} after line 3 ... to $\mathbf{10^{-65}}$ after line 8.

From a detached perspective, no question about the empirical meaning of the results remains. Predictions were consistently correct; with high degrees of certainty. The conjecture, 'Positions of *grahas* cannot influence micro-organism growth rates', stands refuted. The opposite assertion: 'Positions of *grahas* influence growth rates', is not refuted. It requires investigation in more detail in further experimental programs to find out exactly how they do so.

8.4 Scientific Discoveries

Returning from logical and statistical technicalities to common sense language, let us consider the results from a more positive perspective. What do they reveal about growth processes in microbiology? Or about biology itself? Particularly in light of Chapter 7's theory? What do they identify about *grahas'* influence in biology? The discoveries were of three kinds.

First Scientific Discovery: The foremost discovery was that *Jyotisha* concepts were supported:

1. *Jyotisha Muhurtha*: starting time exerts an ongoing influence on a biological process.
2. *Jyotisha* correctly predicts differences between outcomes:
   - Of the *Jyotisha* predictions ('conjectures') tested, *none* were refuted.
3. For starting times when *Guru* exerted an influence, cells grew, or survived, better.
4. Similarly, the North Node of the moon, *Rahu,* was observed to oppose the life of cells.
   - *Rahu*'s influence slowed the growth of cells, but
   - Enhanced propagation of viruses
   - *Rahukala* starting times rendered immune response ineffective.
5. The planet Saturn, *Sani,* decreased immune response; vaccination was less successful.

6. When *Chandra*, the Moon, is in different *Rashis*, she exerts different effects. If strong,
   - *Chandra* supports organisms' growth, and
   - protects them from *Rahu.*

The effects of *Guru, Sani* and *Rahu* were predicted at the outset. Those of *Chandra* were *post-hoc,* observed in the first bacterial growth experiment; identified by correlating days on which the data indicated high growth with days when *Chandra* was strong. They were quantified by 2-Factor ANOVAs and MANOVAs. The second bacterial experiment confirmed that *Chandra* exerts effects lasting an entire day, not just during one rising sign.

Second Scientific Discovery: Supposedly 'auspicious' and 'inauspicious' starting times were observed to exert consistently ***opposite effects*** on outcomes of microbiological processes. Furthermore, such effects were ***opposite*** for bacterial growth and virus propagation. Compared to neutral times, 'auspicious' starting times ***enhance*** bacterial growth and ***reduce*** virus propagation; 'inauspicious' starting times have the ***opposite*** effect, ***reducing*** bacterial growth and ***enhancing*** virus propagation! Special 'inauspicious' times included days of solar eclipses, and *Rahukala.* Experiments testing these ***consistently observed similar effects,*** with eclipses producing a *stronger* effect, exactly as posited by *Jyotisha.*

Third Scientific Discovery: Concerning microbiological processes themselves. The reason, or a large part of the reason for the huge variability observed in many microbiological processes is the starting time. High variances were seen in all processes investigated. IAH&VB scientists know well that, every time they start a vaccine production process, they do not know whether it will be successful or not. Data in Table 4.1 amply illustrates the dangers that they face: only 12 production processes out of forty produced usable BQ vaccine; good quality sporulation is essential. Those not understanding *muhurtha* effects must think *C. Chauvoie* wretchedly capricious bacteria. But that is not the case at all. They appear to require the support of *Guru* or *Chandra* to sporulate successfully! Possibly, a major biological discovery?

In the case of immune response: its high variability is well-known; on average far less than 100%. Flocks need to be vaccinated several times to achieve the 80-90% protection required. Any scientific means to consistently improve levels of immune response would be a boon to the farming and food industries, as well as of fundamental scientific importance. Experiments building on the data obtained in the vaccination experiments could well achieve that advance.

Comment: The sequence of the 3 major discoveries is important. The first two have more certainty: influence of starting time on process outcome is undeniable; 'auspicious' and 'inauspicious' times exert *consistent* influences predicted by *Jyotisha,* meriting comment: experiments on pathogenic bacteria observed the same effects in two different systems; those on virus systems found decreased production under 'auspicious' influences, but *increased* virus production under the other 'inauspicious' influence; the four BT virus experiments produced consistent results. Little doubt can remain about their authenticity, or their opposite natures.

Now consider their implications: in all cases, statistical tests indicated that the data contained interpretable information. If an experiment produces a high F value, then an observation of some phenomenon has occurred. If, as here, a previously unknown and unsuspected effect is being observed, significant values of Fisher's 'F' statistic imply more: *the new effect should be interpreted in the context of known scientific phenomena.* Known theories should be extended, or a new theory should be formulated. Chapter 7 showed how that may be achieved.

8.5 Theory

An important corollary of starting time dependence of microbial growth processes is that it refutes the only present theory, the 'Stochasticity Hypothesis' of complexity scientists, Nina Federoff and Walter Fontana. Apparently random variations in rates are observed in many biological processes. The 'stochasticity' theory suggests that such variations are due to the presence of 'Small Numbers of Large Molecules' in rate-determining steps, which cause key chemical growth processes to be subject to large, purely random variations.

The experiments refute that conjecture entirely. They render the hypothesis null and void. The variations in cellular growth seen in Table 4.1 and Table 4.2 would require those processes in all cells in the same suspension to consistently show the same variations for the same starting time slot. That is against the spirit of the Federoff-Fontana conjecture. *Random* processes in different cells must vary independently of each other; large *random* variations in processes in individual cells must statistically average out to far smaller variations when millions of different cells are involved. Statistically the magnitude of the variations will decrease by the square root of the number of cells. A million cells will reduce the magnitude of the variations by a factor of 1,000, and more as the cells multiply and their numbers increase. This statistical analysis refutes Stochasticity as applied to growth processes *ab initio,* without needing the experiments to do so.

But the ANOVAs add another dimension, adding empirical weight to the theoretical statement: Purely random, 'stochastic', variations in processes involved in bacterial growth and virus propagation could never correlate with values of well-defined external variables, like time of the day, or day of the week. No ANOVA analysing their relationship would ever obtain statistically significant results. Hence, the observed variances in the data *cannot* be due to purely *random* variations in internal microbiological processes. Stochasticity stands refuted.

Proceeding one theoretical step further: high ANOVA 'F' values produce their own challenges. They suggest that some mechanism is at work, enabling external factors to influence micro-organisms' internal processes. The F values challenge us to suggest physics, by which positions of *grahas* may affect the observed processes. Chapter 7 outlined such a theory: suggesting that high levels of quantum correlations internal to *grahas,* created during their condensation at the birth of the solar system, can exert such effects on cellular and organism process regulation, *if regulation is located at criticality.* But, according to studies in complexity biology, location of regulation at criticality is a universal law of biology.

Means by which *grahas* influence processes in microbiology have thus been identified. The conjectured applications of *Jyotisha* astrology to microbiology have gained theoretical support. More work is needed to explain their two kinds of directional dependence: one associated with *graha* positions and their relative dispositions, and the second associated with the positions of the *Rashis,* the orientation of the *Kalapurusha.* Such theoretical possibilities require much further work, but are already under way. The possibility of other, interfering influences should also be considered, as should alternative possible explanations, before they can be ruled out.

8.6 Implications for Jyotisha Astrology

All the experimental results supported *Jyotisha* predictions. Applications of *Jyotisha* did not distinguish one organism from another. They applied to all biological processes and organisms tested, especially processes in single cells. The experiments tested *Jyotisha* predictions for BT virus propagation in baby hamster kidney (BHK21) cells, growth of bacteria, *C. Chauvoie* (anaerobic), and *P. Multocida* (aerobic), and two kinds avian virus propagation.

In all cases, cell growth or resistance to pathology, was tested at times considered auspicious and inauspicious for life. Statistically significant, consistent results obtained throughout, yielding the highly significant **p** values listed in Table 8.1. Cumulative **p** values from all the experiments combined to yield the unheard of statistical significance of $\mathbf{10}^{-65}$.

The results suggest that *grahas* are always influencing biological functions. They reject with a good degree of confidence the materialist position that *no such influences are possible. Jyotisha* influences apparently produce powerful effects in the life of everyone. Chapter 7's theory suggests that *all cells in all organisms are under their influence.* The *Navagrahas* are constantly influencing all organisms.

Now relax from these scientific assertions. Look around you at the plants in your home, office or library. Gaze outside at the living creatures in your environment. Look at them in any picture, photograph, painting or media presentation. The message of the experiments is that *every process in every cell that you see is, in all likelihood, being continuously influenced by the **Jyotisha** grahas.* All processes are regulated from ***criticality***. Every process can be influenced by ***internal quantum correlations*** carried by the *Navagrahas.* That is the message of this book.

Many have realised the intense inspiration of that message. At a WAIRCO technology conference in Colombo, the first author presented a paper on how to apply the experimental results to improve output from vaccine production processes. He made such an impression that he won 'Best Paper in Conference' award. Potential technological applications to industrial microbiological processes were clear to all. The certificate is shown in Figure 8.1.

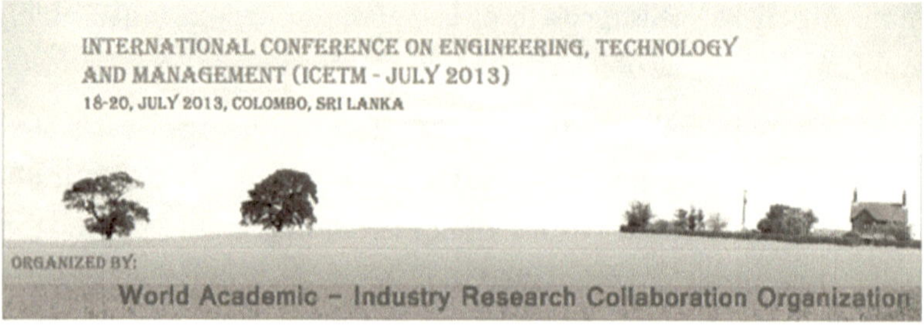

FIGURE 8.1 BEST PAPER IN CONFERENCE AWARD
WAIRCO ICETM Conference, Colombo, 20 July 2013

Date: 20th July 2013

Best paper award in ICSTM – Aug 2013

This is to certify that the below papers were awarded as the best papers presented in the *"International Conference on Engineering, Technology and Management (ICSTM – Aug 2013)"* held during 18-20, August 2013 at Colombo, Sri Lanka. They were awarded to register their paper in the future conference to be held at either in Kuala Lumpur, Malaysia /Hong Kong, China without paying registration fee. If they fail to register in the either of the above conference, this will not be extended further. For more information about the WAIRCO conference, you can visit:

http://www.worldairco.org/Conferences.html .

The papers awarded as best paper are:

S. No. Paper id Name & Address

1 18 Dr. Ramesh Rao N, Assistant Director, Dept. of

Animal Husbandry and Veterinay Services, Govt.

of Karnataka, Bangalore, India

2 23 Mrs. Kumudavalli M V, Dept. of MCA (BU), DSI,

Bangalore, India.

With Best Regards,

C Lakshmikanth

President, World Academic – Industry Research Collaboration Organization (WAIRCO)

http://www.worldairco.org

Epilogue

THE NATURE OF TIME

Starting time, *Muhurtha*, appears to exert non-homogeneous effects on processes later in their development. In all the experiments, time acted as a *heterogeneous* variable. This seems to contradict every assumption made about time in theoretical science; it may seem opposed to the structure of science itself. But Chapter 7 proposed a physical theory suggesting how *grahas* influence complex biological systems, giving time seemingly *heterogeneous* qualities. The physical theory applies to phenomena governed by 'criticality' in complexity biology, especially to phenomena with large variances observed in fractal physiology. Experiments 3, 4 and 6 in Table 8.1 with their 2-Factor ANOVAs demonstrated that substantial fractions of their variances depend on starting time variables. For this reason, the new phenomena need not be considered outside the present body of scientific knowledge. They are universal. They include ALL biological phenomena.

For time immemorial, *Jyotisha* has guided society, rooted in the hearts of those who accepted it without hard scientific evidence. Today is the time to remedy this defect. Precious treasures lie in nature's time-space coordinates, where all phenomena may be observed, and which can be boons for mankind, if they are explored. The growing epidemic of Non-Communicable Diseases makes it urgent to identify new systems of variables. Science only works through sense organ-based understanding. Beyond it, a huge treasury of ancient knowledge awaits.

This work sheds light on one of the most challenging aspects of modern microbiology, the variations in rates of complex processes under close biological regulation: Bacterial Growth; Virus Propagation; and Immune Response. Results suggest that 50-80% of all such variance should be attributed to *Jyotisha* parameters like *Muhurthas*, lunar angle, *graha* positions, strengths, and locations in different houses; all used to discern a person's nature and their qualities of subtle energy.

Understanding these mysteries, we may respect and embrace Nature's Administration. We become dumb before the magnitude and magnanimity of the cosmic administration. Such inner silence can lead us to become instruments in the hands of the Divine. Body, Mind and Soul come into alignment and relax totally; minimal basal metabolic rate and expenditure of subtle energy allow Nature's *Purusha* Administration to take firm control over the natural vagaries of the mind, *Prakriti*.

We have further pointed to explanations in terms of these experiments: the coordination of Nature's alphabet in terms of the chemical elements, and such counterparts in variable events of Absolute consciousness. How it generates different biomolecules, regulated under the genetic loop system governed by different 'frequencies', corresponding to the seven colours, attributable to various *Jyotisha* conditions in the *Janmakundali*: the *Lagna balam, Nakshatra balam*, and the strengths of the Sun and Moon, working on body and mind. All these influence outcomes of regulatory processes, affecting the rate of production of various biomolecules, their size, shape, and patterns, interacting with circadian rhythms and other biorhythms. These are expressed in terms of languages of time: the weekly cycle, the lunar cycle, the cycles of the seasons, the *Ayana,* six-monthly cycle, the annual cycle, and further cycles of Jupiter, the 18.6-year cycle of the lunar nodes, *Rahu* and *Ketu,* and the 60-year *Samvathsara* cycle of Jupiter and Sani combined. States of all such 'frequencies' colour each instant of time.

Overall, the changing nature of each given instant of time means that Nature is in constant flux, influenced by all *grahas,* the permutations and combinations of which affect the outer and inner nature of each body, mind and soul differently. That is why *Jyotisha* knowledge of time and space dimensions is required to assess each person's journey in life.

As we go deeper and deeper into the microworld understanding, we lose our identity in understanding the science of the whole, which depends on the continuous interplay of regulatory processes of an infinitely subtle nature. The interplay is a continuous process of creating new molecules and new compositions of organisms' tissues and cells. The quality of each organ and organ system is constantly being updated by movements in the Heavenly Mansions. These subtle secrets of Nature have been transmitted through the Great Masters who transcended the various space and time domains to arrive at the source of cosmic knowledge, expressed in the ancient Vedic sciences.

One truth should no longer be ignored: time is a subjective research variable, complementing space as an objective variable. Where the two meet and jointly operate, they create new dimensions at each instant of time.

Appendix

CONCEPT OF ENVIRONMENT ACCORDING TO VEDAS: *VĀSTU*

Deeply related to the science of *Jyotisha* is the Vedic science of *Vāstu,* its science of planning within the environment, architecture, building construction and layout. For us humans, our principle environments are our homes and places of work, and the cities where we dwell. Optimizing these for each person is laid out in *Sthapatya Veda,* the Vedic science of architecture, also known as *Vāstu Vidya. Vāstu* concerns ideal siting of a home or work place, within its land and wider environment; the building's internal layout, and specific uses of its various rooms or other parts. *Vāstu's* texts describe principles of ground preparation, spatial organization and sizes in relation to the owner's physique and *Jyotisha Janmakundali,* and other aspects of overall design and layout. *Vāstu-Vidya* explains how such factors exert subtle influences on the lives of those who dwell in them, particularly, but not restricted to, their health and longevity. *Vāstu* principles include those for design and layout of houses, shops, temples, gardens, roads, water works, and public areas of towns and cities.

Vāstu can also be seen as an application of *Jyotisha* to diagrams, in objective language. It explains the qualities of energy in an enclosed space or cavity. It explains that energies in different directions or orientations in the interior and exterior of the cavity have different qualities of subtle energy, labelling these qualities with one or other of the *Grahas,* planets. Its designs integrate architecture with nature, using symbolic *yantra* patterns to determine functions of various regions of an overall structure according to compass directions. A *yantra* behaves as a physical template acting on a subtle level, generating and maintaining subtle energies supporting a person's life-force, as identified by their *Jyotisha Janmakundali.*

From this perspective, *Vāstu* is a science of the *pancha mahabhutas,* showing how their subtle influences affect spatial elements in the different parts of an architectural design, and how the effects of its cavity structure influence different people. The *Vedas* explain how different directions are commanded by the subtle energies of the different *grahas.* Like all Vedic sciences, *Vāstu's* concern is thus with influences at subtle levels. Every enclosed space, or 'cavity', holds an internal distribution of subtle energies. *Vāstu* offers a knowledge of cavity systems that accords to each direction in space a subtle energy identified with one of the *Jyotisha grahas* (see Figure 2). A close relationship thus exists between the two sciences, *Jyotisha* and *Vāstu*: *Jyotisha* makes recommendations for a person's ideal *Vāstu.*

Like all the ancient sciences, *Vāstu Vidya* and *Jyotish* work on the principle that the manifest world of sensory experience is built up in layers, and that underlying the gross realm of sensory experience, there are levels of subtle experience that only become available when awareness is refined, and sensitivity has developed on levels that are *sukshma* or subtle. Indeed, the ability to interact on subtle sensory levels is one of the main purposes of traditional practices taught by the ancient Vedic *Rishis* to their children, described in such stories as those of *Brighu* and *Svetaketu* in the *Taittiriya* and *Chandogya* Upanishads.

Figure 2: Planetary Qualities of the Eight Directions in *Vāstu*

North-West **Chandra – Moon**	**North** **Buddha – Mercury**	**North-East** **Guru – Jupiter** **Ketu – South Node**
West **Sani – Saturn**	**Brahmasthana** **Surya – Sun**	**East**
South-West **Rahu – North Node**	**South** **Mangal – Mars**	**South-East** **Shukra – Venus**

The central idea in all Indian sciences is that each subtle level controls the level above it. Learning to operate on subtle levels of nature is therefore the key to gaining control of different aspects of life. This can even be seen in western life, since the Vedic sciences regard the intellect as subtler than the mind, and in control of its content. Those with higher intellects tend to find themselves acknowledged as sources of inspiration, knowledge and expertise for others needing guidance in various fields.

In the case of human life itself, the Vedic Sciences name various 'subtle bodies' that control the *annamayokosha,* the gross physical body acknowledged by modern bioscience: the *pranamayokosha* (or body of vital energy), the *manomayokosha* (or body of mind including feelings and emotions), the *vijnanamayokosha,* or body of higher intellect with knowledge of the subtle realms, and the *anandamayokosha,* or body of deep spiritual experience and understanding.

www.ingramcontent.com/pod-product-compliance
Lightning Source LLC
Chambersburg PA
CBHW030908180526
45163CB00004B/1760
9781647836436